Anish Manocha
Suresh D.K.
Rajvir Malik

Bone Morphogenetic Proteins

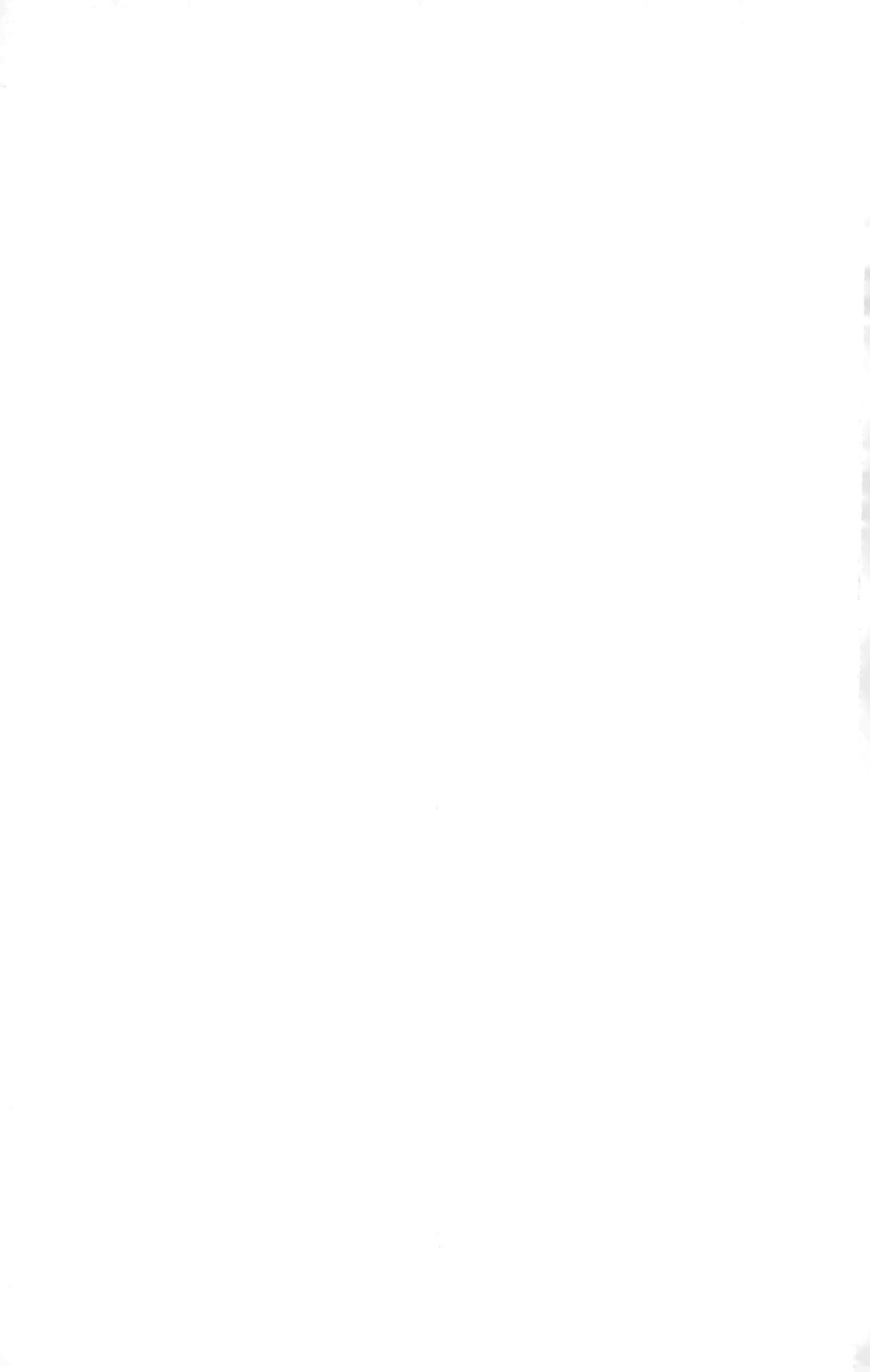

Anish Manocha
Suresh D.K.
Rajvir Malik

Bone Morphogenetic Proteins

A Potential Stimulant in Bone Regeneration

LAP LAMBERT Academic Publishing

Impressum/Imprint (nur für Deutschland/only for Germany)
Bibliografische Information der Deutschen Nationalbibliothek: Die Deutsche Nationalbibliothek verzeichnet diese Publikation in der Deutschen Nationalbibliografie; detaillierte bibliografische Daten sind im Internet über http://dnb.d-nb.de abrufbar.
Alle in diesem Buch genannten Marken und Produktnamen unterliegen warenzeichen-, marken- oder patentrechtlichem Schutz bzw. sind Warenzeichen oder eingetragene Warenzeichen der jeweiligen Inhaber. Die Wiedergabe von Marken, Produktnamen, Gebrauchsnamen, Handelsnamen, Warenbezeichnungen u.s.w. in diesem Werk berechtigt auch ohne besondere Kennzeichnung nicht zu der Annahme, dass solche Namen im Sinne der Warenzeichen- und Markenschutzgesetzgebung als frei zu betrachten wären und daher von jedermann benutzt werden dürften.

Coverbild: www.ingimage.com

Verlag: LAP LAMBERT Academic Publishing GmbH & Co. KG
Heinrich-Böcking-Str. 6-8, 66121 Saarbrücken, Deutschland
Telefon +49 681 3720-310, Telefax +49 681 3720-3109
Email: info@lap-publishing.com

Herstellung in Deutschland (siehe letzte Seite)
ISBN: 978-3-659-13069-4

Imprint (only for USA, GB)
Bibliographic information published by the Deutsche Nationalbibliothek: The Deutsche Nationalbibliothek lists this publication in the Deutsche Nationalbibliografie; detailed bibliographic data are available in the Internet at http://dnb.d-nb.de.
Any brand names and product names mentioned in this book are subject to trademark, brand or patent protection and are trademarks or registered trademarks of their respective holders. The use of brand names, product names, common names, trade names, product descriptions etc. even without a particular marking in this works is in no way to be construed to mean that such names may be regarded as unrestricted in respect of trademark and brand protection legislation and could thus be used by anyone.

Cover image: www.ingimage.com

Publisher: LAP LAMBERT Academic Publishing GmbH & Co. KG
Heinrich-Böcking-Str. 6-8, 66121 Saarbrücken, Germany
Phone +49 681 3720-310, Fax +49 681 3720-3109
Email: info@lap-publishing.com

Printed in the U.S.A.
Printed in the U.K. by (see last page)
ISBN: 978-3-659-13069-4

Copyright © 2012 by the author and LAP LAMBERT Academic Publishing GmbH & Co. KG and licensors
All rights reserved. Saarbrücken 2012

CONTENTS

	CHAPTER NAME	PAGE NO.
1)	Introduction	03 – 04
2)	Bone Morphogenetic Proteins	05 – 06
3)	Historical Perspective	07 – 13
4)	Structure and Classification	14 – 17
5)	Functions of BMP	18
6)	Mechanism of Action	19 – 25
7)	Signalling Mechanism	26 – 33
8)	Carriers of BMP	34 – 50
9)	Tissue Regeneration	51 – 71
10)	Dosimetry	72 – 74
11)	Release Kinetics	75 – 77
12)	Immunogenicity	78 – 81
13)	Future trends	82 – 86
14)	Summary and Conclusion	87 – 88
15)	Appendix – 1 (Abbreviations)	89 – 90
16)	References	91 – 113

ACKNOWLEDGEMENT

To begin with, I thank the most merciful and compassionate, the **ALMIGHTY GOD.**

It is my privilege and honour to acknowledge and express my sincerest gratitude to my mentor, **Dr. SURESH D.K.,** M.D.S., Professor and Head, Department of Periodontology, M.M. College of Dental Sciences and Research, Mullana, for his advice, supervision and crucial contribution. His involvement with his originality has nourished my intellectual maturity that I will benefit from, for a long time to come.

I express my deep sense of gratitude to **Dr. RAJVIR MALIK,** Professor, Department of Periodontology, D.A.V. Dental College, Yamunanagar, Harayana for his valuable guidance, constructive suggestions, and encouragement. He is a constant oasis of ideas and passions in dentistry, which exceptionally inspire and enrich my growth as a student and a researcher.

My parents deserve special mention for their inseparable support and prayers. My Father, **Sh. ASHOK MANOCHA**, showed me the joy of intellectual pursuit ever since I was a child. He has supported me thoughout with his exemplary guidance, unlimited encouragement and undying spirit in igniting the flame of knowledge in me. My Mother, **MRS. ANITA MANOCHA,** is the one who sincerely raised me with her care and gentle love. It is because of their love, care, confidence and support that brought out the best in me. I hold them in high esteem. Words fail me to express my appreciation for my sister**, Ar. ADITI MANOCHA** whose dedication, love and persistent confidence in me, has taken the load off my shoulder.

Dr. ANISH MANOCHA

CHAPTER 01

INTRODUCTION

> *" Science is the most exciting and sustained enterprise of discovery in the history of our species. It is the great adventure of our time.*
>
> *We live today in an era of discovery that far outshadows the discoveries of the New World five hundred years ago."*
>
> <u>Michael Crichton</u>

Bone is a living, dynamic tissue with substantial capacity for regeneration. Since the advent of tissue engineering, bone has received particular interest, since it is one of the tissues with most regenerative abilities in the human body.

Marshall Urist *discovered that non living demineralised bone could become fully mineralised living functional bone when implanted at ectopic sites, and he coined this phenomenon* **"bone by auto-induction"**.[1] He hypothesised that the principle behind this regenerative potential resides in the extracellular matrix of bone and termed it **"Bone Morphogenetic Proteins (BMPs)"**.

Bone morphogenic proteins (BMPs) are a group of growth factors and cytokines known for their ability to induce the formation of bone and cartilage. They represent a unique set of differentiation factors that *induce new bone formation at the site of implantation instead of changing the growth rate of pre-existing bone*. Given that BMP's induce new bone growth, in vivo, promote the recruitment and growth of osteoblast progenitor, and maintain the expression of osteoblast phenotypes in cultures, it is conceivable that providing *an optimal dose of a BMP in the circulation may help trigger the osteogenic responses, as an endocrine signal, and restore the loss of bone mass and quality.*

Bone morphogenetic proteins (BMPs) are multi-functional growth factors that are structurally related to transforming growth factor beta (TGF - β) superfamily and activins, and are responsible for migration, proliferation and differentiation of several cell types.[2] The roles of BMPs in embryonic development and cellular functions in postnatal and adult animals have been extensively studied in recent years. BMPs also play an important role in postnatal bone formation. BMP activities are regulated at different molecular levels.

BMPs have promising potential for clinical bone and cartilage repair, working as powerful bone-inducing components in diverse tissue-engineering products **(Reddi - 1998, 2005)**[3-4]. *BMP's are the first therapeutic proteins approved for the use of tissue engineering in conjuction with a scaffold and biocompatible fixative devices in the arena of regenerative medicine*[5].

Synthetic polymers, natural origin polymers, inorganic materials and composites may be used as carriers for the delivery of BMPs. Carriers range from nano-particles to complex three-dimensional (3D) scaffolds, membranes for tissue-guided regeneration, biometric surfaces and smart thermosensitive hydrogels.

Current clinical uses include spinal fusion, healing of long bone defects and craniofacial and periodontal applications. *BMP-2 and BMP-7 have recently received approval by the US Food and Drug Administration (FDA) for specific clinical cases, delivered in absorbable collagen sponges.* Considering the expanding number of publications in the field of BMPs, there are prospects of a brilliant future in the field of regenerative medicine with the use of BMPs.

CHAPTER 02

BONE MORPHOGENETIC PROTEINS

Rh - BMP (recombinant bone morphogenetic protein) is a genetically engineered protein which recruits bone forming cells to the surgical area and "turns on" local cells to the bone-making process. BMP is used for stimulation of bone growth.

In the initial experiments done by **Marshall Urist**[1] almost 50 years ago, he was able to identify a mixture of proteins isolated from the bone marrow, which were activated when the bone was damaged. It was not until the late 1980's that the individual protein components could be separated and identified. The tests used to determine the relative potency of the individual protein components involved placing a small amount of the material beneath the skin of test animals. *Some, specifically rhBMP-2, were able to stimulate immature local mesenchymal (soft-tissue) cells to become bone forming cells.*

The finding was both an amazing scientific discovery and a warning. Consider the possibilities of a material that could alter the way a body forms bone and heals itself. *If BMP placed under the skin could turn tissues to bone, what about the nearby blood vessels and nerves? What if they also turned to bone? Think of the possibilities for injury.* The key to controlling this powerful material involves understanding the mechanisms that are involved in the stimulation and regulation of bone formation. The difficulty for surgeons is knowing where and how to place the material so that bone forms in the correct places, but does not form in areas which could injure the patient.

Also, there are basically two reasons to use BMP instead of the patient's own bone. First, the animal studies and the preliminary human studies show a higher and more successful fusion rate from BMP when compared to patients own bone. That means that the likelihood of a solid fusion occurring and the bones healing together properly is better when the surgeon uses BMP.

The second reason is that by using BMP the surgeon does not have to take any patients own bone. When the marrow or cancellous bone is taken from the patient's bone there is always some additional pain and blood loss. It may be minimal, but it still requires additional surgery. The site where the bone is taken from (donor site) has a risk of long-lasting pain, infection, and nerve damage as well. It simply makes the most sense to use BMP since it provides a higher fusion rate with a lower risk of complications and less surgery.

CHAPTER 03

HISTORICAL PERSPECTIVE

In the early 1960s, several researchers were investigating the process of calcification. In a series of experiments designed to test his *triphasic theory of calcification*, **Urist and co-workers** discovered that control samples of untreated decalcified bone implanted into muscle pouches of rabbits and rats resulted in new cartilage and bone formation. This led to the hypothesis of *bone formation by autoinduction,* in which an inductor cell (a *"wandering histiocyte"*), acts upon an induced cell (a fixed histiocyte or peri vascular young connective tissue cell), causing it to differentiate into either an osteoprogenitor or a chondroprogenitor cell (**Van de Putte & Urist 1965, 1966, Urist 1965, Urist et al. 1967, Urist 1994**)[1,6-10.] However, *Urist was not the first to allude to this theory of bone formation by autoinduction, or of the hypothetical bone-inducing substance which he later referred to as "bone morphogenetic protein."*

In 1938, **Levander**[11] reported on a series of experiments designed to study bone regeneration. Initially, he implanted living bone fragments 1 to 1.5 cm in length either subcutaneously or intramuscularly. These fragments were first treated by scraping away the periosteum, and in some specimens a superficial layer of bone was also removed.

Upon obtaining regenerated bone, Levander was able to show that it was neither the periosteum nor cells on the surface or within the graft that were responsible for new bone growth. *Since it was evident that new bone was formed from the mesenchymal tissue which surrounded the graft, he proposed that there must be some stimulating agent which originated from the graft itself, possibly a substance which was soluble in the lymph tissue.*

In subsequent experiments, alcoholic extracts of bone were injected intramuscularly, resulting in 22% of sites forming cartilage or bone, 80 controls received injection of alcoholic solutions of similar concentration and volume, resulting in no cartilage or bone development.

Levander thus concluded that there is an extractable substance from bone which is able to activate mesenchymal cells to form bone tissue. He also reasoned that this is the most likely explanation for bone formation in muscle tissue after trauma, as well as the possibility that this substance circulating in the blood may be the cause for other types of heterotopic bone formation (**Levander 1938**)[11].

Lacroix 1945[12] reported results from experiments using implanted cartilage as well as alcoholic extracts from the cartilaginous epiphyses of the long bones of rabbits, and concluded that the observed bone formation was due to an induction phenomenon and originated from a substance or a group of substances within the cartilage which he suggested calling ***osteogenin.***

A few years later, **Heinen et al** [13] challenged the hypothesis of a specific osteogenetic substance as proposed by Levander, Lacroix and others. In an effort to substantiate the findings of Levander, *Heinen discovered that a number of animals developed bone and cartilage following an injection of alcohol alone.* Further investigations with other irritating substances and conditions without the use of alcoholic extracts of bone revealed a number of interesting findings.

The amount of ectopic bone and cartilage formation was increased by exercising the animals, and larger amounts of bone and cartilage were formed in younger animals as compared to older ones.

Heinen concluded that this hypothetical osteogenetic substance could not be proved, and stated that it was unfortunate that investigations studying this hypothesis had used mainly *the rabbit, a species which "has manifested a high incidence of ectopic cartilage and bone in many organs following a wide variety of experimental procedures."*

ISOLATION OF BMP

Even though Urist was not the first to speculate on the existence of a bone inducing substance, he must be credited with much of the early work involved in the isolation of bone morphogenetic protein (BMP). Not knowing specifically how or what to look for led to many years of experiments resulting in much information in regards to methods and procedures in obtaining positive results of bone formation but little information as to what specifically was causing this bone induction to take place. As previous investigators reported conflicting results over the use of decalcified bone matrix to fill surgical bony defects.[14]

It was realized that in order to properly assess the bone inducing capacity of an implant of demineralised bone, the implant must be placed away from orthotopic bone either subcutaneously or in muscle pouches.[10] Many animal species were tested with implants of demineralized bone which was prepared using a variety of chemical agents with respect to temperature, concentration and time.

In reviewing their own observations as well as previous literature on decalcified bone matrix, **Van de Putte and Urist** *realized that implants of bone decalcified in either nitric acid or ethylenediaminetetra- acetic acid (EDTA) generally led to negative results, and bone decalcified in hydrochloric acid led to positive results.*

Bone matrix decalcified in nitric acid produced an intense inflammatory reaction, rapid disintegration of the implant, and no new bone formation.[10] Implants of bone demineralised in low concentrations of EDTA at 4°C and a neutral pH produced limited bone formation in rats or rabbits, but none in guinea pigs or dogs (**Urist & Strates 1971**)[15]. Bone decalcified in cold (2°C) dilute (0.6N) HCl for less than 3 to 5 days, followed by washing in 0.15M NaCl or 70% alcohol produced the most positive results. Modifications of this method of preparation helped to bring into focus components within bone which contained the bone morphogenetic property.

By the late 1960s, evidence was established that the substance which was responsible for bone induction was intimately associated with bone collagen. However, it was still uncertain whether the inducing property was due to a specific chemical or if the physical structure of collagen itself was in some way directing the mechanism for mesenchymal cell differentiation (**Urist et al 1968**)[16]. Speculation as to the location or substance responsible for the morphogenetic activity focused on the quaternary and inter fibrillar cross links of collagen (**Urist et al 1968**)[16], telopeptides of the non-helical region of collagen (**Urist & Strates 1971**)[15] and/or a non-collagenous protein bound to bone collagen (**Urist et al, 1972**)[17].

A later study (**Syftestad & Urist 1979**)[18] revealed that pulverization of bone particles to less than 44 µm led to inactivity of the bone morphogenetic property most likely due to free radical formation from energy absorption and molecular chain rupture, both leading to protein denaturation. These studies helped to confirm that the *osteo-inductive property in bone matrix was the result of a non collagenous bone morphogenetic protein.*

TRANS-MEMBRANE DIFFUSION

Pulverization of bone matrix was found to inactivate the inductive substrate, initially supposed either through denaturation of the protein structure (**Urist & Dowell 1968**)[16] or by changing the geometry of the bone matrix (**Reddi & Huggins 1973**)[19]. An experiment designed to test the morphogenetic activity of various sizes of bone particles used preparations of bone matrix pulverized in a freezer mill at -199°C in order to minimize the possible protein damage resulting from heat (**Urist et al 1977**)[20]. Diffusion chambers made up of cellulose acetate membranes having a thickness of 150 μm and pore size of 0.45 μm were also used for the purpose of determining whether the physical characteristics of the particles themselves were an important factor or if inactivity observed with smaller particles was a factor of rapid diffusion and disappearance of the inductive substrate before the cells capable of mixing induced could arrive. Diffusion chambers from 1 to 5 membranes thick were used for the experimental implants. Control implants were placed outside of the membranes. In the controls, particle sizes of 400-1000 μm resulted in new bone formation, while 75-149 μm and 44-74 μm particles produced no new bone.

In single-walled chambers, 44-74 μm particles produced no new bone. However, in double-walled chambers, half of the test sites produced transmembrane osteogenesis. It was also shown that with the larger particle size of 400-1000 μm, the amount of new bone formation on the outside of the membranes decreased from the closest membrane to the farthest.

Therefore, the amount of new bone formation was shown to be inversely proportional to the distance which the bone morphogenetic property must travel. This experiment provided evidence of a rapidly diffusible bone morphogenetic property when previously none was believed to exist (**Urist & Dowell 1968**)[16].

By retaining this diffusible property through multiple walled chambers even the smaller particles which are more soluble and therefore disintegrate faster were able to induce new bone formation, A later study (**Syftestad & Urist 1979**)[18] revealed that pulverization of bone particles to less than 44 μm led to inactivity of the bone morphogenetic property, most likely due to free radical formation from energy absorption and molecular chain rupture both leading to protein denaturation. *These studies helped to confirm that the osteoinductive property in bone matrix was the result of a noncollagenous bone morphogenetic protein.*

PURIFICATION

Isolation and purification of BMP has been difficult due to the fact that so little of it is present in bone as compared to other non collagenous proteins, and also because of its relative insolubility. However, by the early 1980s, methods which utilized large quantities of bone and a number of steps to separate out different fractions of the non collagenous proteins yielded a group of low molecular weight components which proved positive for bone induction (**Urist et al, 1982, Mizutani & Urist 1982, Urist et al 1984**)[21-23].

Briefly, frozen cortical bone was ground to a particle size of 1 mm^3 demineralized in 0.6 N HCl at 4°C for 48 h, then defatted in 1:1 chloroform methanol. Using different concentrations of $CaCl_2$ or GuHCl and urea, the noncollagenous proteins were extracted from the insoluble bone matrix gelatin and separated into different fractions, Subfractionation was then accomplished using ultrafiltration. SDS gel electrophoresis and various types of chromatography in order to determine which molecular weight components were responsible for BMP activity.

Early studies indicated that the molecular weight of bovine BMP was in the range of 12 kD to 30 kD with strong evidence for a BMP of 17 to 18 kD (**Urist et al, 1982, Mizutani & Urist 1982**)[21]. In order to determine which fractions or subfractions were capable of inducing bone formation, a reconstitution assay was utilized, this most commonly being accomplished in the rat (**Sampath & Reddi 1981**)[24]. The protein to be tested was reconstituted with collagenous bone matrix which was devoid of endogenous BMP and then implanted subcutaneously. The formation of bone indicated a positive response to the implanted protein.

Major advancement in the field of BMP research took place when **Wang et al**[25] through SDS-polyacrylamide gel electrophoresis identified a group of proteins from bovine bone of 30 kD (after reduction i.e. in monomeric form, they were 16, 18 and 30 kD) and then proceeded to isolate recombinant clones for each. Amino acid sequences of the 16, 18 and 30 kD components were used to develop probes to screen bovine cDNA libraries. The matching recombinant clones obtained were then used to screen the corresponding human cDNA libraries. Thus, recombinant human proteins BMP 1, BMP 2A and BMP 3 were obtained and their biochemical and biological characteristics including amino acid sequences revealed (**Wozney et al 1988**)[26].

Soon afterwards isolation and characterization of five additional BMPs (BMP 4 through BMP 8) was carried out with BMP-2A and BMP-2B now being called BMP-2 and BMP-4 respectively (**Wozney 1989, Wozney et al, 1990, Celeste et al, 1990**)[27-29]

CHAPTER 04

STRUCTURE, FORMS & CLASSIFICATION

Bone morphogenetic proteins are members of TGF superfamily, a large family of growth factors. *The TGF was so named because of its ability to transform cultured fibroblasts.* There are several structural homologies between BMPs and TGF growth factors. The amino acid sequence of BMPs is highly conserved and is considered to be as old as 600 million years. Because of this conservation human recombinant BMPs are highly effective in lower life forms including fruit flies.

Like all members of the TGF family, BMPs are synthesized as precursor proteins. The precursor protein contains hydrophobic secretive leader sequence as well as substantial pro-peptides. *The mature portion of the protein is located at the carboxy terminal of the precursor molecule. In their carboxy terminal portions, all BMPs contain seven cysteine amino acid residues in positions identical to those present in all members of the TGF superfamily.* In addition, BMPs contain N-linked glycosylation sites.

Of all the BMPs thus far reported in the literature, BMP-2 through BMP-9 are related to one another. Also due to their amino acid sequences, BMP-2 through BMP-9 are classified as belonging to the TGF-β superfamily. Like other members of the TGF- β superfamily, they are derived from precursor polypeptide chains ranging in size from 396-513 amino acids **(Wozney 1994)**[30]. Each precursor is made up of an N-terminal secretory leader sequence and a highly conserved C-terminal region containing 114-139 amino acids **(Ripamonti & Reddi 1994)**[31]. It is the amino acid conservation in the C-terminal region including a series of seven completely conserved cysteine residues which characterize the members of the TGF- β superfamily.

An exception to this involves BMP-8, which contains an 8th cysteine in this region **(Ripamonti & Reddi 1994)**[31].

The mature active BMP molecule is derived from the carboxy terminus portion of the precursor chain and like other members of the TGF-β family, it is expected to be in the form of a dimer. *Whether the BMPs exist only as homodimers is unknown.* Other members of the TGF-β family are known to exist as heterodimers **(Massague 1990)**[32].

BMP 2 through BMP 8 can be divided into 3 subgroups based on similarities in their amino acid sequences.

- BMP 2 and BMP 4 form one group having 92% amino acid identity within the seven cysteine domain of the mature region.
- BMP 5 through BMP 8 form a second group having 82% identity in this region. These 2 subgroups have 59% homology with one another and only 45% homology with BMP 3 which forms a group by itself **(Wozney 1995a)**[33].
- BMP-9 has 50-55% homology with BMPs 2, 4, 5, 6 and 7 **(Song et al 1995)**[34].

As part of the TGF-β superfamily, the BMPs are related to other proteins (dpp, Vg 1, etc) critical to differentiation and developmental processes during embryonic development. In addition to their role in embryonic development, BMP 2 through BMP 8 have also been shown to induce cartilage and bone formation in the post fetal model.

TGF-β in its various forms is similar to the BMPs in that it is actively expressed throughout embryonic development and into adulthood **(Thompson et al 1989)**[35]. TGF-β has also been shown to have growth stimulatory effects on bone **(Joyce et al 1990)**[36].

However, the BMPs are the only known molecules capable of forming cartilage and bone in an ectopic site. It is interesting to note that the BMPs share more sequence homology with some of the other proteins in the superfamily than with TGF- β1, β2 and β3. Overall amino acid sequence homology within the C-terminal region between all members of the TGF- β superfamily ranges from 25 to 80% **(Burt 1992)**[37].

The *Drosophila* dpp protein, important in dorsal-ventral specification during embryogenesis is closely related to BMP 2 and BMP 4 having about 75% amino acid sequence identity to both. It has been suggested that one of these BMPs is the human homolog of the dpp protein **(Wozney et al, 1988)**[25].

BMP-2 and BMP-4 are "highly conserved derivatives of a gene which was present in an ancestor common to the arthropod and vertebrate lineages" **(Gelbart 1989)**[38].

Other members of the TGF- β superfamily include :
- Vgr 1 - a gene product expressed during embryogenesis in the mouse and which is homologous to BMP 6 **(Lyons et al, 1989, Wozney 1992)**[39-40].
- Growth differentiation factors (GDF) 5, 6 and 7 which form a subgroup of BMP-related factors **(Storm et al 1994)**[41].
- The Mullerian inhibiting substances (MIS) which causes regression of the Mullerian duct during male sexual differentiation.
- The *Xenopus* Vg I - a gene product spatially restricted to the vegetal pole of the egg.
- The inhibins and activins implicated in follicle stimulating hormone release by pituitary ceils **(Massague (1990)**[32].

Osteogenin, a molecule purified from bovine bone is the bovine equivalent of BMP 3 **(Luyten et al 1989)**[42]. *BMP 6 is the human homolog of murine Vgr-1. BMP-7 and BMP-8 are also known as Osteogenic Protein OP-1 and OP-2 respectively.*

BMP 1, because of its amino acid sequences cannot be classified as belonging to the TGF-β3 superfamily. It is not capable of inducing bone formation. However, it does have an amino acid sequence similarity with a crayfish protease, a sequence similarity to epidermal growth factor and may have some synergistic effects with the other BMP molecules **(Wozney et al. 1988)**[26].

Homologies of BONE MORPHOGENETIC PROTEIN family members (C-terminal domain)	
	%identity
Drosophila dpp	100
Human BMP – 2	74
Human BMP – 4	76
Human BMP - 3(osteogenin)	43 (with dpp)
Drosophila 60A	100
Xenopus Vg-1	50
Human BMP – 5	72
Human BMP - 6 (murine vgr-1)	71
Human OP- 1 (BMP - 7)	69
Human OP- 2 (BMP - 8)	65

CHAPTER 05
FUNCTIONS OF BMP'S

BMP	FUNCTION
BMP - 2	Osteoinductive, Osteoblast differentiation and apotosis.
BMP - 3	Inhibits Osteogenesis and is most abundant BMP in bone.
BMP - 4	Osteoinductive, promotes eye and lung development.
BMP - 5	Helps in Chondrogenesis.
BMP - 6	Helps in Chondrogenesis and osteoblast differentiation.
BMP - 7	Osteinductive, helps in development of eye and kidney.
BMP - 8	Osteoinductive.
BMP - 9	Hepatogenesis and helps in development of nervous system.
BMP - 10	Helps in cardiac development.
BMP – 11	Helps in neuronal tissues development.
BMP – 12	Induces tendon and iliac tissue formation.
BMP – 13	Induces tendon and ligament tissue formation.
BMP – 14	Enhances tendon healing and bone formation.
BMP – 15	Modifies follicle stimulating hormone activity.

CHAPTER 06

MECHANISM OF ACTION

By using somatic cell hybrid lines and cDNA hybridization probes, BMPs 1 through 7 have been mapped to the following human chromosomes:

- BMP-1 to chromosome 8;
- BMP-2 and BMP-7 to chromosome 20;
- BMP-3 to chromosome 4, further sublocalized to 4pl4-q21;
- BMP-4 to chromosome 14;
- BMP-5 and BMP-6 to chromosome 6 **(Tabas et al. 1991, Hahn et al, 1992, Tabas et al. 1993)**.[46-48]

BMP FAMILY IN HUMANS AND CHROMOSOME LOCATION

BMP Subfamily	Genetic Name	BMP Designation	Chromosome Location
BMP 2	BMP - 2A	BMP – 2	20
BMP 4	BMP - 2B	BMP – 4	14
BMP 3	Osteogenin	BMP – 3	4
	Growth differentiation factor -10 (GDF-10)	BMP - 3B	10
OP-1 / BMP 7	BMP -5	BMP - 5	6
	Vegetal related -I (Vgr-1)	BMP - 6	6
	Osteogenic protein -1 (OP-1)	BMP - 7	20
	Osteogenic protein -2 (OP-2)	BMP - 8	-
	Osteogenic protein -3 (OP-3)	BMP - 8A	-
Others	BMP —9	BMP - 9	-
	BMP -10	BMP - 10	-
	Growth differentiation factor - 11	BMP - 11	-
CDMP	Cartilage-derived morphogenetic protein-1 (CDMP-1) / Growth	BMP - 14	20
	Cartilage-derived morphogenetic protein-2 (CDMP-2) / Growth	BMP - 13	-
	Cartilage-derived morphogenetic protein-3 (CDMP-3) / Growth	BMP - 12	-
Others	BMP- 15	BMP - 15	-
	BMP – 16	BMP - 16	-

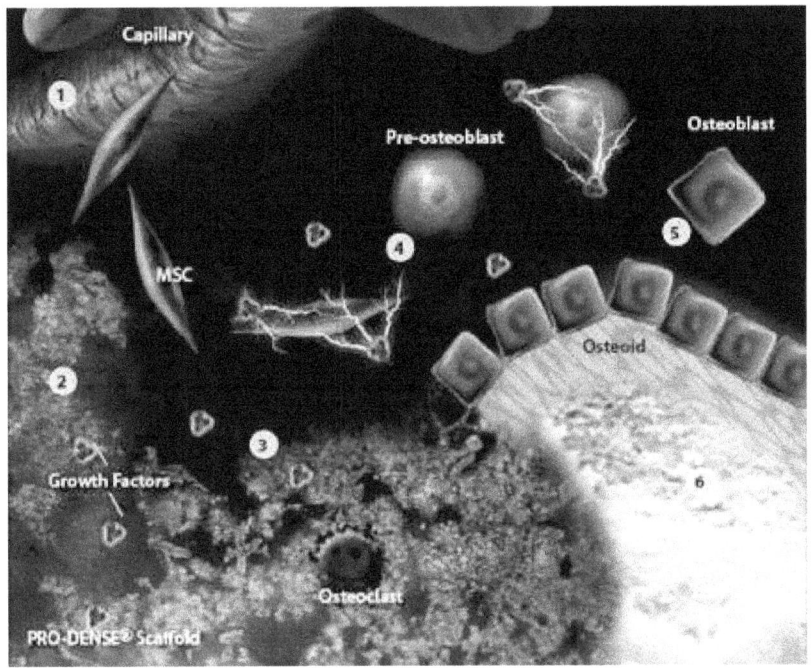

Proposed Mechanism of Action [54]

1) Angiogenesis is a key early event. The $CaSO_4$ of the implant resorbs first, revealing a porous calcium phosphate scaffold conducive to vascular infiltration.
2) The resulting brushite/TCP scaffold with interconnecting pores binds free proteins such as VEGF and BMP-2 at the implant/defect interface.†
3) Resorption of the PRO-DENSE® scaffold releases bound proteins. Active proteins recruit cells to the implant surface.†
4) Growth factors in the implant/defect interface region, including BMPs, stimulate proliferation and differentiation of mesenchymal stem cells.
5) Differentiated osteoblasts lay down osteoid which then mineralizes to become newly woven bone.
6) The principles of Wolff's Law drive remodeling.

BONE MORPHOGENETIC PROTEINS – SPECIFIC ANTAGONISTS

Recent work has also identified Bone Morphogenetic proteins – specific antagonists and member of the DAN family. The members of DAN family mCer1, gremlin and several genes that only been identified as sequence tags.

> - These antagonists bind to the Bone Morphogenetic proteins with the same affinity as Bone Morphogenetic proteins receptors do. Local irradiation also inhibits Bone Morphogenetic proteins induced bone formation. An over expression or dysregulation of Bone Morphogenetic proteins pathwaysmay lead to heterotropic bone formation or fibroplasias ossificans progressive (FOP). Bone Morphogenetic proteins have been implicated in FOP. The pioneering work of Sakou has implicated Bone Morphogenetic proteins in ossification of the posterior longitudinal ligament of the spine in Japnese patients.

> - The Bone Morphogenetic proteins – specific antagonists such as noggin or chordin might be used therapeutically in clinical conditions with pathologically excessive bone formation.

BONE INDUCTION CASCADE

- Bone induction by demineralised bone matrix is a multistep cascade.
- The major phases of osteoinduction are chemotaxis, mitosis and differentiation.
- Chemotaxis may be defined as the directional migration of the cells in response to a chemical gradient. Implantation of demineralised bone matrix promotes chemotaxis of cell to the vicinity. Plasma fibronectin binds avidly to the implanted bone matrix[55]. Fibronectin is a protein with a molecular mass of 450

Kd and has affinity for collagen, fibrin, and heparin. It is well known that peptides of fibronectin are chemotactic and perhaps mitogenic.
- The next major phase of bone induction is mitosis. Proliferation of newly attached mesenchymal cells indicates that the bone matrix is a local mitogen. The mitogenic action can be quantified by measuring DNA synthesis, using radio autography and isotope incorporation.
- The mitotic phase is followed by the differentiation of cartilage, vascular invasion and bone differentiation.
- By day 3, most leukocytes have disappeared and numerous elongated fibroblast like mesenchymal cells appear in close proximity to the implanted matrix and proliferate. There was no evidence of phagocytosis of matrix material by fibroblasts. It would appear that matrix cell interaction results in the transformation of mesenchymal cells into chondroblasts on day 5.
- Numerous chondrocytes are present on days 7 to 8.
- With the advent of capillary invasion on day 9, chondrocytes hypertrophy and the first signs of mineral formation evident in matrix of hypertrophied chondrocyte.
- By days 10 and 11, numerous multinucleate chondroclasts appear close to the regions of chondrolysis. Concurrently, osteoblasts with intense basophilia appear close to the vascular endothelium and new bone is formed by appopositional growth on the surface of the calcified matrix and the implanted non living collagenous matrix. Multinuclcatc ostcoclasts with the characteristic ruffled border remodel the newly formed bone by days 12 to 18, resulting in selective dissolution of implanted matrix and the formation of an ossicle consisting essentially of the newly induced bone.
- Between days 16 and 21, there is further remodelling of bone marrow elements, including erythrocytic and granulocytic series and megakarocytes.

TIME AFTER IMPLANTATION	CELLULAR EVENTS	MOLECULAR PROCESSES
1 MIN	* Blood clot formation * Platelet release	*Fibrin network formation. *Release of platelet derived growth factors. *Binding of plasma fibronctin to implanted matrix.
1 hour	*Arrival of PMN by chemotaxis	*Release of proteolytic enzymes such as collagenase and elastase
18 hours	*Accumulation of PMN's * Adhesion of cells	*Limited proteolysis and release of chemotactic factors for fibroblasts.
Day 1	*Chemotaxis of fibroblasts & Cell attachment to implanted extra cellular matrix	*Release of peptide of fibronectin increased cell motility. *Role of microtubules and microfilaments
Day 2	*Continuation of chemotaxis for fibroblasts. *Signal transduction from matrix to cell surface.	*Initiation of protein and nucleic acid synthesis. *Release of growth factors.
Day 3	*Cell Proliferation	*Thymidine incorporation into DNA * Increase in ornithine decarboxylase activity
Day 5	*Differentiation of Chondroblasts	*Increase in SO_4 incorporation into proteoglycans.
Day 7	*Chondrocytes synthesis and secretion of matrix	*Type II collagen synthesis, cartilage specific Proteoglycans
Day 9	*Hypertrophy of chondrocytes *Calcification of cartilage matrix *Vascular invasion	*Increase in Ca incorporation and alkaline phosphatise activity. *Type IV collagen synthesis, Laminin and factor VIII in blood vessels.
Day 10-12	*Osteoblasts bone formation and mineralisation	*Type I collagen synthesis. *Bone proteoglycans synthesis. *Peak in Ca incorporation and alkaline phosphatise activity.
Day 12-18	*Osteoclasts bone remodelling and dissolution of implanted matrix.	*Increase in lysosomal enzymes. *Upswing in accumulation of y-carboxyglutamic acid containing protein. *Release of collagenases and proteases.
Day 21	*Bone marrow Differentiation	*Increase in Fe incorporation into heme. *Accumulation of lysozyme.

BIOCHEMICAL CHANGES

- Mesenchymal cell proliferation on day 3 is quantitated by measuring the amount of H-thymidine incorporation into cellular DNA and the activity of ornithine decarboxylase in the implant.

- Induction of new cartilage is quantitated by sulphate incorporation into cartilage specific proteoglycans and immunpfluroscent localisation of type II collagen[56-57].

- The appearance of bone and the mineralisation of this newly induced bone is indicated by an increase in the specific activity of alkaline phosphatase and Ca incorporation into bone mineral from day 9 onward.

- Determing the elevated levels of lysosomal enzymes acd phosphatase and arylsulphatase in day 14 implants monitors bone remodelling.

- The differentiation of hematopoitic marrow is accompanied by an increase in the incorporation of iron into heme[57].

CHAPTER 07

SIGNALLING MECHANISM OF BMP

- The BMP receptors on the cell surface are made up of Type I and Type II serine / threonine kinase proteins.
- Kinases are enzymes that phosphorylate proteins called Smads and activate them.
- The binding of the ligand to the Types I and II serine/threonine kinase transmembrane receptors results in the formation of hetero-tetramer complex and activation of the signaling cascade.
- Immediately after the binding, the Type II receptor kinase phosphorylates the Type I receptor.
- In turn, the Type I receptor phosphorylates the intracytoplasmic signaling molecules Smads 1, 5, and 8.
- There are eight different Smads. Smads 1,5 and 8 are substrates for Bone Morphogenetic proteins receptors.
- Smads 2 and 3 are substrates for TGF-β and activin receptors.
- Phosphorylation of Smad 1,5 and 8 activates it to interact with common functional partner Smad 4, and this heteromeric complex enters the nucleus to active turn on Bone Morphogenetic proteins – responsive genes.
- There are two inhibitory smads 6 and 7, that normally reside in the nucleus and act as a relay to inhibit or turn off Bone Morphogenetic proteins type I receptor kinase – mediated phosphorylation of Smads 1, 5 and 8.
- Thus, there is an intricate homeostatic regulation of the Bone Morphogenetic proteins receptor – activated turning on genes and their turning off by Smads 6 and 7 through the inhibition of type I Bone Morphogenetic proteins receptor kinase phosphorylation.

LIGAND BINDING

The TGF Beta superfamily of ligands include:

- *Bone morphogenetic proteins (BMPs),*
- *Growth and differentiation factors (GDFs),*
- *Anti mullerian hormone (AMH),*
- *Activin, Nodal and TGF β.*

Signalling begins with the binding of a TGF beta superfamily ligand to a TGF beta type II receptor. The type II receptor is a serine/threonine receptor kinase, which catalyses the phosphorylation of the Type I receptor. Each class of ligand binds to a specific type II receptor[58]. In mammals there are seven known type I receptors and five type II receptors[59].

There are three activins:

Activin A, Activin B and Activin AB.

Activins are involved in embryogenesis and osteogenesis. They also regulate many hormones including pituitary, gonadal and hypothalamic hormones as well as insulin. They are also nerve cell survival factors.

The BMPs bind to the Bone morphogenetic protein receptor type-2 (BMP-R2). They are involved in a multitude of cellular functions including osteogenesis, cell differentiation, anterior/posterior axis specification, growth, and homeostasis.

The TGF β family include:

TGF-β1, TGF-β2, TGF-β3.

Like the BMPS, TGF β's are involved in embryogenesis and cell differentiation, but they are also involved in apoptosis, as well as other functions. They bind to TGF-β receptor type-2 (TGFBR-2).

Nodal binds to activin A receptor, type IIB ACVR2B. It can then either form a receptor complex with activin A receptor, type IB (ACVR1B) or with activin A receptor, type IC (ACVR1C)[59].

RECEPTOR RECRUITMENT AND PHOSPHORYLATION

The TGF β ligand binds to a type II receptor dimer, which recruits a type I receptor dimer forming a hetero-tetrameric complex with the ligand[60]. These receptors are serine/threonine kinase receptors. They have a cysteine rich extracellular domain, a trans-membrane domain and a cytoplasmic serine/threonine rich domain. The GS domain of the type I receptor consists of a series of about thirty serine-glycine repeats.

The binding of a TGF β family ligand causes the rotation of the receptors so that their cytoplasmic kinase domains are arranged in a catalytically favorable orientation. *The Type II receptor phosphorylates serine residues of the Type I receptor, which activates the protein.*

SMAD PHOSPHORYLATION

There are five receptor regulated SMADs:

SMAD-1, SMAD-2, SMAD-3, SMAD-5, and SMAD-9 (sometimes referred to as SMAD-8).

There are essentially two intracellular pathways involving these R-SMADs.

- TGF β's, Activins, Nodals and some GDFs are mediated by SMAD-2 and SMAD-3.
- BMPs, AMH and a few GDFs are mediated by SMAD-1, SMAD-5 and SMAD-9.
- The binding of the R-SMAD to the type I receptor is mediated by a zinc double finger FYVE domain containing protein.

Two such proteins that mediate the TGF β pathway include

- *SARA (The SMAD anchor for receptor activation)* and
- *HGS (Hepatocyte growth factor-regulated tyrosine kinase substrate)*

SARA is present in an early endosome which, by clathrin-mediated endocytosis, internalizes the receptor complex[61]. SARA recruits an R-SMAD. SARA permits the binding of the R-SMAD to the L 45 region of the Type I receptor[62]. SARA orients the R-SMAD such that serine residue on its C-terminus faces the catalytic region of the Type I receptor. The Type I receptor phosphorylates the serine residue of the R-SMAD. Phosphorylation induces a conformational change in the MH2 domain of the R-SMAD and its subsequent dissociation from the receptor complex and SARA[63].

CoSMAD binding

The phosphorylated RSMAD has a high affinity for a coSMAD (e.g. SMAD4) and forms a complex with one. The phosphate group does not act as a docking site for coSMAD, rather the phosphorylation opens up an amino acid stretch allowing interaction.

TRANSCRIPTION

- The phosphorylated RSMAD/coSMAD complex enters the nucleus where it binds transcription promoters/cofactors and causes the transcription of DNA.
- Bone morphogenetic proteins cause the transcription of mRNAs involved in osteogenesis, neurogenesis, and ventral mesoderm specification.
- TGF β cause the transcription of mRNAs involved in apoptosis, extracellular matrix neogenesis and immuno-suppression. It is also involved in G1 arrest in the cell cycle.
- Activin causes the transcription of mRNAs involved in gonadal growth, embryo differentiation and placenta formation.
- Nodal causes the transcription of mRNAs involved in left and right axis specification, and mesoderm and endoderm induction.

PATHWAY REGULATION

The TGF β signaling pathway is involved in a wide range of cellular process and subsequently is very heavily regulated. There are a variety of mechanisms that the pathway is modulated both positively and negatively. There are agonists for ligands and R-SMADs; there are decoy receptors; and R-SMADs and receptors are ubiquitinated.

(a) Following ligand binding to a pre-formed hetero-dimeric receptor consisting of one BMPR type II (BMPR-II) and one BMPR-I, BMPR-II phosphorylates BMPR-I; activated BMPR-I in turn phosphorylates BMP-restricted Smads (R-Smads: Smad-1, 5 and -8), which, once phosphorylated (P-Smads), form a complex with the common-partner Smad (Co-Smad: Smad-4), to translocate to the nucleus and regulate gene transcription.

(b) However, if ligand binding leads to recruitment of receptors to a complex consisting of one BMPR-II and homo-oligomerised BMPR-I, subsequent BMPR-II phosphorylation of BMPR-I might lead to activation of mitogen-activated protein kinases (MAPKs), including p38, in certain cell types.

LIGAND AGONISTS / ANTAGONISTS

Both chordin and noggin are antagonists of BMP's. They bind BMP's preventing the binding of the ligand to the receptor. It has been demonstrated that Chordin and Noggin dorsalize mesoderm. They are both found in the dorsal lip of *Xenopus* and convert otherwise epidermis specified tissue into neural tissue. Noggin plays a key role in cartilage and bone patterning. Mice Noggin have excess cartilage and lacked joint formation[64].

Members of the DAN family of proteins also antagonize TGF β family members. They include Cerberus, DAN, and Gremlin. These proteins contain nine conserved cysteines which can form disulfide bridges. *It is believed that DAN antagonizes GDF-5, GDF-6 and GDF-7.*

Follistatin inhibits Activin, which it binds. It directly affects follicle-stimulating hormone (FSH) secretion.

Follistatin also is implicated in prostate cancers where mutations in its gene may preventing it from acting on activin which has anti-proliferative properties[64].

RECEPTOR REGULATION

The Transforming growth factor receptor 3 (TGFBR 3) is the most abundant of the TGF-β receptors yet, it has no known signaling domain[65]. It however may serve to enhance the binding of TGF β ligands to TGF β type II receptors by binding TGF β and presenting it to TGFBR 2.

One of the downstream targets of TGF β signalling, *GIPC*, binds to its PDZ domain, which prevents its proteosomal degradation, which subsequently increases TGF β activity. It may also serve as an inhibin co-receptor to Activin RII.

BMP and Activin membrane bound inhibitor (BAMBI), has a similar extracellular domain as type I receptors. It lacks an intracellular serine/threonine protein kinase domain and hence is a pseudo-receptor. It binds to the type I receptor preventing it from being activated. It serves as a negative regulator of TGF β signaling and may limit TGF β expression during embryogenesis. It requires BMP signalling for its expression.

R-SMAD regulation

Role of inhibitory SMADs

There are two other SMADs which complete the SMAD family, the inhibitory SMADs (I-SMADS), SMAD-6 and SMAD-7. They play a key role in the regulation of TGF β signalling and are involved in negative feedback. Like other SMADs they have an MH1 and an MH2 domain. SMAD-7 competes with other R-SMADs with the Type I receptor and prevents their phosphorylation[66]. It resides in the nucleus and upon TGF β receptor activation translocates to the cytoplasm where it binds the type I receptor. SMAD-6 binds SMAD-4 preventing the binding of other R-SMADs with the coSMAD.

The levels of I-SMAD increase with TGF beta signaling suggesting that they are downstream targets of TGF-beta signaling.

R-SMAD ubiquitination

The E3 ubiquitin-protein ligases SMURF1 and SMURF2 regulate the levels of SMADs. They accept ubiquitin from a E2 conjugating enzyme where they transfer ubiquitin to the RSMADs which causes their ubiquitination and subsequent proteosomal degradation. SMURF-1 binds to SMAD-1 and SMAD-5 while SMURF 2 binds SMAD-1, SMAD-2, SMAD-3, SMAD-6 and SMAD-7. It enhances the inhibitory action of SMAD-7 while reducing the transcriptional activities of SMAD-2.

BONE MORPHOGENETIC PROTEIN (BMP) SIGNAL TRANSDUCTION.

Smad and TGF-beta1 Activated tyrosine Kinase 1 (TAK1). The Smad pathway is induced by the phosphorylation by type I receptor of an intracellular protein called Receptor-regulated Smad (R-Smad). Two phosphorylated R-Smad molecules form a complex with a Common-partner Smad (Co-Smad). This complex is translocated into the nucleus and interacts with transcription factors (TF) to activate target genes transcription. The Smad signal pathway is regulated by Inhibitory Smad (I-Smad) that binds to type I receptors.

CHAPTER 08

CARRIERS FOR BMP

Bone morphogenetic protein is a water-soluble relatively low-molecular weight protein that diffuses very easily in the body fluids. When administered in a surgical setting, the protein will diffuse very rapidly in wound hematomas or can be irrigated away or lost in the suction drainage, henceforth, it is necessary to contain the BMP. In an experimental setting BMP delivered without a carrier does not endure more than a few hours at the deposited site. *It is therefore necessary to contain the BMP in a carrier so that it will have a localized effect at the bone healing site.*[67]

The need for a carrier has been recognized since BMP was initially identified. Various carriers have been investigated experimentally and clinically. The BMP carriers can be broadly classified into *inorganic salts, naturally occurring polymeric substances, synthetic polymers, and composites of synthetic and naturally occurring polymers.*

CHARACTERISTICS OF AN IDEAL CARRIER[68]

- An ideal carrier should neither induce an inflammatory response nor immune reaction.
- Degradation of the carrier should not result in toxic residues.
- Ideally the carrier should be absorbed concurrent with bone healing, leaving no residue.
- It should be porous, the porosity being equivalent to cancellous bone.
- The carrier should protect the BMPs from degradation and maintain its bioactivity while releasing the protein in a time and space controlled way to promote the formation of new bone at the treatment site.

- Carriers should be conveniently sterlizable, easy to handle, stable over time with well-defined storage procedures, as well as suitable for commercial production, allowing scale-up production and approval by regulatory agencies.

The porosity permits trapping of inflammatory cells and bone growth factors. Debate exists regarding the ideal configuration and the sizes of the porosity needed for bone growth. There are competing claims concerning the intercommunicating nature of the porosity with open ends at the surface and the size of the pores. It is generally agreed that the pore size should be at least comparable with the porosity in the cancellous bone. Pore size even larger than that is thought to be beneficial. Whether the pores should be blind pockets or communicating with each other as well as with the environment is somewhat debatable, and there is no definitive answer to this question.

PROPERTIES OF CARRIER :

1) *Osteoconductivity of the carrier*
Grafts with good osteoconductive properties form a tight bond with the host tissue, which is desirable for the restoration of the bone function at short notice. The osteoconductivity of DBM, which mainly consists of collagen type I, has been well shown[69]. Most synthetic materials containing hydroxyapatite also show good osteoconductive properties. Bioactive glasses and synthetic ceramics support the bonding of bone tissue. The bioactive glasses form a tight bond with tissue through the HCA layer that is formed on the glass surface after implantation[70,71]. Polymers are not osteoconductive, but a combination of hydroxyapatite with polymers into a composite was found to improve the graft-to-bone binding[72].

2) Bioactivity of carriers

Several carriers for BMPs have shown distinct osteogenic properties by themselves, which may be supportive for BMP-dependent osteoinduction. Collagen type I has been shown to stimulate osteoblastic differentiation of cells in culture[73]. *In vivo*, the addition of collagen type I was shown to aid bone formation in grafts containing osteogenin[74]. PGLA implanted in the medullary canal in sheep stimulated local osteogenesis[75]. *In vitro*, PGLA stimulated growth and osteogenic differentiation of osteoblastic cells[76]. Hollinger[77] found an accelerated rate of healing of tibial defects in rats after grafting with a co-polymer of PLA and PGA. The osteogenic effects of ceramics and bioactive glasses are often ascribed to the binding of native proteins and growth factors to the surface of these grafts. The local accumulation of extracellular factors at the glass surface may subsequently stimulate, or even induce, bone formation[78].

3) Biocompatibility of carriers

Titres of antibodies against allogenic or xenogenic implants of collagen have been reported occasionally, but did not show interference with bone formation at the grafted site[79]. However, collagen of allogenic or xenogenic origin causes a potential risk of pathogen transmission[80]. Synthetic carriers should be free of this risk, but rejection or unwanted tissue reactions can still occur. Inflammatory tissue reactions have been reported after implantation of Phydroxyapatite-polymers [81,82] and resorbable ceramics, but addition of BMP seems to decrease the inflammatory reaction. Zegzula and colleagues[83] showed that increasing the amounts of BMP-2 on a co-polymer carrier caused a decrease of inflammatory cell infiltrate.

It is not clear whether the inflammatory reaction is a wanted or an unwanted side effect. Inflammatory cells release cytokines, which may mediate the bone formation process. Indeed, enhanced BMP dependent bone formation, probably mediated by interleukin-1, was seen in mice with a systemically induced inflammation. However, it is well known that *chronic inflammation as a result of, for example, periodontitis or rheumatoid arthritis, stimulates bone resorption and is not a desirable condition for bone induction*[84].

4) *Geometry of the carrier*

The geometrical properties of a carrier may greatly influence the performance of the BMP graft. *Geometrical parameters such as size and shape can influence the degradation rate of the carrier, the rate of release of BMP, and the bonding of bone to the implant.* Some geometrical configurations, for example solid hydroxyapatite particles and solid polymer discs, have been found to be unfavourable for bone induction[89]; conversely, *porous discs or blocks of hydroxyapatite were favourable for bone induction,* and granules of hydroxyapatite with identical pore dimensions did not elicit bone formation. Pore size of hydroxyapatite was found to be optimal between 300–400 mm.

Sigurdsson and coworkers[90] have shown that the *consistency of the BMP-loaded carrier also determines the extent of the area where bone is formed and its density.* They reported that use of bovine tendon-derived type I collagen and PGLA co-polymer carriers resulted in a high bone density, but a low total bone volume, because these carriers were not able to maintain the defect space adequately. DBM and bovine crystalline bone matrix did maintain the defect space adequately, resulting in a larger bone area, but lower bone density.

5) *Kinetics of release of BMP from a carrier*

BMPs in solution are quickly cleared from the system, which may explain why very high doses of BMP are needed for bone induction when they are used without a carrier. An appropriate carrier retains BMP at the grafted site for a period of time sufficient to induce bone. The kinetics of release of the BMP from the carrier and the retention of biological activity of BMPs are of crucial importance to successful bone induction. *A too rapid clearance of BMP is effectively prevented by the use of collagen carriers.* Release studies show that collagen carriers release a bulk of BMP initially, followed by a more gradual release thereafter. This release pattern is effective, but the question remains whether the dose of BMP can be further decreased and retain a more sustained release pattern.

Combination of BMPs with non-resorbable ceramics did not result in bone induction[85]. This is probably due to the lack of resorption of hydroxyapatite and the strong binding of BMPs to hydroxyapatite, which prevents BMP release. Indeed, *when BMPs were combined with resorbable ceramics, bone was induced*[86]. When non-resorbable ceramics were combined with BMPs and collagen, bone induction was not hindered, possibly because of a sufficient release of BMP from the collagen[85].

Polymers and bioactive glasses are promising materials for drug delivery, as their material properties – and thus their release kinetics – can be varied by changing the production procedure or the ratio of their components. However, a matter of concern with these carriers is that a large proportion of the proteins do not retain activity after release from the carrier.

6) *Biodegradation of carrier*

Carrier degradation after implantation is preferable, in order to aid the release of BMP and to obtain complete replacement of the graft by bone. Bioactive glasses and PLA/PGA polymers degrade after contacting (body) fluids, whereas degradation of collagen and resorbable ceramics does not depend on cellular activity. *When the degradation is too slow, bone formation can be inhibited*[87]*; when the degradation is too fast, BMPs are released too rapidly and the risk of fibrous ingrowth, and thus failure of bone healing, is increased.* Biodegradation of the carrier should therefore coincide with the rate of endogenous bone formation. Addition of BMP to a carrier affects the resorption rate of the carrier. An enhanced resorption rate of PLA and DBM carriers in the presence of BMP has been observed in several studies[88].

CARRIER BMPS

1) Synthetic biodegradable polymers

Synthetic polymers have been widely used in tissue engineering applications (**Saito and Takaoka, 2003**)[91]. Initially, polylactic acid (PLA) was investigated as a carrier for BMP delivery (**Miyamoto et al, 1992**)[92] but the material was considered ineffective due the release of acidic degradation by-products. However, novel biodegradable synthetic polymers have attracted attention, since these are free of the risk of disease transmission that occurs with other materials used for bone applications, such as collagen. Biodegradable polymers, such as polylactic acid–p-dioxanone–polyethylene glycol (PLA–DX–PEG), allow percutaneous injection after heating, for use as a scaffold and a delivery carrier for BMPs, due to its versatile temperature-dependent liquid–semisolid transition. This plasticity allows the biodegradation of the polymer to be synchronized with the induction of new bone by BMP, and this type of injectable polymeric delivery system, polymerization *in situ*, enables a less invasive approach to bone surgery (**Saito et al, 2003**)[93].

In other reports, composites of PLA–DX–PEG with calcium phosphate were shown to require less rhBMP to induce new bone formation in mice (**Matsushita et al, 2004**)[94] and in healing femur defects of rabbits. Composites of PLA–PEG with hydroxyapatite were also evaluated for articular cartilage repair in rabbits and in a rabbit radii model (**Kaito et al, 2005**)[95], showing enhanced tissue repair in the animals treated with rhBMP-2 and hydroxyapatite composites. Polylactic-co-glycolic acid (PLGA) combines the adsorptive stability of PLA with the mechanical strength of polyglycolic acid (PGA) and has received particular attention (**Winet and Hollinger, 1993**)[96].

Biodegradation of the synthetic composite is achieved by varying the proportion of each of the two component materials. PLGA as a carrier for rhBMP-2 delivery was reported in alveolar cleft repair in dogs **(Mayer et al, 1996)**[97], in gelatine sponge composites in a rabbit ulna model **(Kokubo et al, 2003)**[98], in tooth defects of dogs **(Kawamoto et al, 2003)**[99] and in combination with bone marrow cells in a rabbit segmental bone defectmodel **(Hu et al, 2005)**[100]. These studies confirm the good results that are usually obtained with PLGA scaffolds; bone formation was observed successfully when the scaffolds delivered rhBMP, as compared to controls.

Another report, which involved a PLGA scaffold conjugated to heparin, showed that a much longer sustained release of rhBMP 2 and significantly increased *in vivo* new formation of bone were achieved **(Jeon et al, 2007)**[101], indicating the promising potential that heparin has as a stabilizing agent for BMP bioactivity. Synthetic polymers have been also formulated as hydrogels for the delivery of BMPs. Since hydrogels contain large amounts of water, they are interesting devices for the delivery of therapeutic proteins.

Lutolf[102] reported using synthetic PEG based hydrogels that mimic the invasive characteristics of extracellular matrices, with integrin-binding sites for cell attachment and substrates for matrix metalloproteinases, in a rat model for rhBMP-2 delivery. The authors demonstrated that cells were able to fully penetrate the hydrogels and bone tissue was formed within 3–4 weeks in the gels that delivered rhBMP-2. Similarly, PEG based hydrogels were reported by **Pratt**[103], showing that cells were able to fully invade the gel networks that were conjugated with peptides that mimic characteristics from extracellular matrix, such as plasmin and a heparin molecule to improve the rhBMP-2 stability.

A major disadvantage of the use of synthetic polymers is the risk of an inflammatory response, due to acidic by-products of degradation, which may be also detrimental to the stability of the incorporated BMPs. This has led researchers to look forward to other materials, such as collagen and other natural polymers, as alternatives for BMP delivery.

2) Collagen

Collagen is the major non-mineral component of bone and also the most abundant protein in connective tissues of mammals. Collagen has received much attention due to having good biocompatibility, degrading into physiologically compatible products and being suitable for interaction with cells and other macromolecules. The large variety of collagen formulations includes collagen gels, demineralized bone matrix, fibril collagen, collagen strips, membranes, absorbable collagen sponges and composites **(Geiger *et al*, 2003)**[104].

Another advantage is that collagen can be processed in aqueous form. *Collagen also has a favourable influence on cell infiltration and wound healing.* During the last years, most researchers have focused on the use of absorbable collagen sponges, although several other formulations have been investigated **(Kirker-Head 2000)**[105]. *Collagen sponges are very versatile, easily manipulated and wettable.* The manufacture of collagen sponge carrier depends on several factors, including sponge mass, cross-linking methods, sterilization methods, soaking time, protein concentration and buffer composition **(Geiger *et al*, 2003)**[104].

For collagen sponges, binding of rhBMP is highly dependent on pH. Studies using modified versions of recombinant BMP led to the conclusion that modification of the isoelectric point could bring up to 100-fold differences in the retention of protein to the collagen carrier. Binding of rhBMP-2 is therefore dependent on the isoelectric point of the two proteins and other factors, such as ionic strength.

Collagen sponges have since been tested and evaluated in several animal models and clinical trials for cases of fracture repair, critical size defects, spinal fusion and dental and craniofacial reconstruction **(Geiger *et al*, 2003)**[104].

The collagen sponge consists of lyophilized rhBMP, which is reconstituted with water prior to injection and impregnates the collagen sponge for several minutes before implantation. Two models using collagen sponges delivering recombinant human BMP-2 or BMP-7 were approved by the FDA for human use as an alternative to bone grafts, for spinal fusion and long bone fractures, after many pre-clinical trials that have been recently reviewed **(Gautschi *et al*, 2007)**[106]. The collagen sponge holds the BMP and releases it only in the local environment where the surgery was performed, eliminating the need to harvest autologous bone, which causes post-operative pain.

Based on the extensive preclinical and clinical trials, the use of collagen sponges delivering BMPs has been revealed to be a safer and superior alternative to autogenous bone grafting. However, although showing success, collagen sponges pose risks of immunogenic reactions, since the collagen used on these applications is derived from animal tissues, creating concerns about the risks of transmission of infectious agents and immunological reactions. For this reason, the development of a superior carrier material for BMP delivery based on other natural polymers is currently being investigated.

Alternatively, other sources of collagen, i.e. of recombinant origin, provides a means of obtaining reliable and chemically defined sources of purified human collagens that are free of animal components **(Yang *et al*, 2004)**[107].

3) Natural origin polymers

The materials for tissue engineering applications should ideally mimic the natural environment of tissues and, in this regard, natural polymers can send signals to guide cells at the various stages of their development and thus accelerate healing **(Mano and Reis, 2007)**[108].

There are several natural polymers that may be used as carriers for BMP delivery. These include *starch-based polymers, chitin and chitosan, hyaluronans, alginate, silk, agarose, soya and alga-derived materials, and polyhydroxyalkanoates* **(Mano et al, 2007)**[108].

Several of these polymers are derived from substances occurring in bone, cartilage or the extracellular matrix. For this reason, these materials often present excellent properties for use in regenerative medicine applications, such as being biodegradable, bioresorbable and versatile, as they may be processed into different formulations **(Malafaya et al 2003)**[109].

Natural polymers may present risks of immunogenic reactions and disease transmission and disadvantages such as the sourcing and processing of the materials. Nevertheless, researchers have been looking for materials from plant origin and produced by microorganisms and/or from recombinant technology which may overcome these concerns.

Alginate is a generally safe polysaccharide, known to support the proliferation of chondrocytes *in vitro*. Very interesting work has been developed by Saito and colleagues with small synthetic peptides corresponding to BMP-2 regions binding to cell receptors, incorporated in cross-linked alginate gels, showing *in vitro* osteogenic differentiation and success in repairing bone defects in rats and in rabbit radial bone defects **(Saito et al)**[93].

The use of alginate seems to be particularly appealing for cartilage tissue-engineering applications, since alginate is a major component of cartilage tissue.

Chitosan is another natural degradable polymer, obtained by alkaline deacetylation of chitin, extracted from the exoskeletons of arthoropods. Chitosan has been formulated in many forms, such as hydrogels and fibre meshes, that showed potential for use in osteochondral tissue engineering, making it suitable for BMP delivery **(Prabaharan and Mano, 2005)**[110].

Several studies have reported the use of chitosan for delivering BMPs, particularly in composites with synthetic polymers or with other natural polymers. A chitosan–alginate composite gel, loaded with mesenchymal stem cells and rhBMP-2, was evaluated as an injectable tissue-engineering construct in mice and induced new trabecular bone formation over a period of 12 weeks. Liang and colleagues described a chitosan–gelatine scaffold with incorporated rhBMP-2 **(Liang *et al*, 2005)**[111] which demonstrated increased expression of bone-marker osteocalcin in osteoblast and myoblast cell lines. In another report, a chitosan blend with PGA was studied as a novel delivery carrier for rhBMP-2 **(Hsieh *et al*, 2006)**[112].

Derivatives of chitosan are also reported. *Chemical modification of chitosan may enhance certain bioactive properties and increase its solubility in water*, thus aiding in the incorporation of rhBMPs, such as in the case of carboxymethyl chitosan.

Recently, rhBMP-2 was immobilized directly on a guided bone-regenerative membrane surface, made of chitosan nanofibres, that functioned as a bioactive surface to enhance bone-healing. The BMP-2-conjugated membrane surface retained bioactivity for up to 4 weeks of incubation, as well as holding over 50% of the initial BMP-2 attached, promoting cell attachment, proliferation, ALP activity and calcification, when compared with BMP-2 absorbed to the membrane.

In two other studies, dextran/gelatine-based microspheres, containing rhBMP-2, were adhered to chitosan films for guided tissue regeneration and chitosan membranes activated with BMP-2 were also reported to successfully differentiate C2C12 cells **(Lopez-Lacomba et al, 2006)**[113].

Fibrin is derived from blood clots and can be formulated into an adhesive glue-like delivery system **(Hattori, 1990)**[114]. Fibrin has been used as a delivery system for BMPs in a variety of animal models, including the use of a fibrin–fibronectin sealing system for rat calvarial defects as a carrier for rhBMP-4 and for rhBMP-2, and a fibrin sealant with rhBMP-2 in the healing of dental pulp of dogs.

In these reports, bone formation was much higher when the fibrin carrier was loaded with the rhBMP, as compared to controls. Fibrin glue might be also a great aid in limiting the diffusion of BMPs into the surrounding tissues, which could cause undesirable biological effects. In a rat spinal model, fibrin glue significantly limited the diffusion of rhBMP-2 that was loaded into a collagen sponge, preventing the BMP from inducing bone growth in the surrounding spinal cord and nerves **(Patel et al, 2006)**[115].

Recently, a study using fibrin constructs to deliver rhBMP-2, vascular endothelial growth factor (VEGF) and fibroblast growth factor-2 (FGF-2), combined with hyaluronic acid or collagen, dramatically improved the ability of blood vessels to directly invade the fibrinbased scaffolds **(Smith et al, 2007)**[116].

Finally, a human trial was reported showing partial reconstruction of a frontal bone defect using heparin together with bovine collagen, hyaluronic acid and fibrin as vehicles for rhBMP- 2 **(Arnander et al, 2006)**[117]. Altogether, fibrin glue certainly seems to be a very useful addition to a bone tissue engineering scaffold using BMPs, considering that it aids in promoting osteoinduction and retention of growth factors.

Hyaluronans are present in the extracellular matrix and can be formulated into gels, sponges and pads. Hyaluronans have been used in a variety of trials as a delivery vehicle for rhBMPs, including in sponge form in the treatment of alveolar ridge defects in dogs, periodontal repair in dogs, in sheep in combination with hydroxyapatite, in the healing of critical size defect in rats in composites with polylactic acid and in gel and paste forms in non-human primates. **Kim and Valentini (2002)**[118] evaluated the kinetics of hyaluronic acid as a delivery system for rhBMP-2 *in vitro* and demonstrated that *hyaluronan-based carriers retained more BMP than collagen gels.*

Recently, a acrylated hyaluronic acid hydrogel was used with human mesenchymal stem cells and rhBMP-2 for healing of rat calvarial defects **(Kim *et al*, 2007)**[119]. Higher levels of osteocalcin expression and bone formation occurred when the BMP-2 and stem cells were tested.

Hyaluronans are observed to interfere positively with BMP cascade **(Zou *et al*, 2004)**[120] and, since these are part of the extracellular matrix, they may well be priority choices as scaffolds for the delivery of BMPs in regenerative medicine of bone.

Gelatine has been used mostly in form of hydrogels for delivery of BMPs. Gelatine is an irreversibly hydrolysed form derived from collagen that is usually cross-linked or hardened through thermal treatment to reduce its high water solubility and enhance the retention of protein to achieve a long-term release.

Gelatine hydrogels delivering rhBMP-2 were studied in rabbit skulls, in mice and recently in the skulls of non-human primates. Gelatine hydrogels delivering rhBMP-2 were observed to show higher levels of ALP and osteocalcin in comparison with rhBMP-2 delivered in collagen sponges.

Recently, thermo-mechanical hydrogels based on methacrylated dextran in combination with gelatine have been reported by **Chen *et al.* (2007)**[121]. The group used rhBMP-2 encapsulated in microspheres of the same materials, loaded into the hydrogels, which delivered the growth factor over a period of 18–28 days.

Dextran is another natural polysaccharide, synthesized by some bacteria, that has attracted attention for use as a BMP delivery system, because of its excellent hydrophilic nature and biocompatibility. Dextran has been particularly used in the form of nanospheres for delivery of rhBMPs. Dextran hydrogels has been evaluated for rhBMP-2 delivery, both *in vitro* and *in vivo*, in a rat ectopic model, showing formation of new bone **(Maire *et al*, 2005)**[122]. The possibility of using natural polymers for designing intelligent hydrogel systems for BMP delivery is also an interesting and very attractive option. However, no studies have been reported with the use of these systems.

Starch-based polymers are another interesting alternative for delivering BMPs that was proposed by Reis as materials with high potential for tissue engineering of bone and cartilage, due to their interesting mechanical properties. These starch-based polymers are used in composites with different synthetic polymers and have been formulated into a variety of forms, such as hydrogels, nanofibres, microparticles or 3D scaffolds.

The wide variety of formulations and composites make these polymers suitable scaffolds for bone tissue engineering and controlled release of BMPs. In general, composites of natural polymers with synthetic polymers may become the future option of choice for bone tissue engineering, since they combine the specificities of synthetic and natural polymers to produce superior materials.

Silk fibroin is a protein derived from cocoons made by the larvae of silkworms. Silk has been proposed and widely investigated as a delivery carrier for BMPs in some contributions reported by the Kaplan group. In one study, rhBMP-2 was directly immobilized on silk fibroin films and the effect of the delivery system studied in human bone marrow stromal cells and in critical-sized cranial defects in mice (**Karageorgiou *et al*, 2004**)[123]. The rhBMP retained its biological activity.

In another report, silk scaffold fibres, prepared by electrospinning, were used to deliver rhBMP-2 and hydroxyapatite nanoparticles for *in vitro* bone formation (**Li *et al*., 2006**)[124]. The rhBMP-2 survived the aqueous-based electrospinning process in bioactive form and induced osteogenesis in cultures of human mesenchymal stem cells.

In both studies, the delivered rhBMP-2 increased levels of ALP activity and calcium deposition and transcript levels for bone sialoprotein, osteopontin and osteocalcin.

In recent years Meinel and co-workers have evaluated the use of silk for tissue engineering constructs with silk–RGD covalently bound matrices, in human mesenchymal cells (**Meinel *et al*, 2004**)[125], but not with use of BMPs. Meinel *et al*. tested human stem cells loaded in silk fibroin scaffolds, in combination with rhBMP-2, and compared stem cells transfected with BMP-2 via an adenovirus with exogenous protein. The expression of osteogenic markers was induced but the BMP was not studied when delivered directly on the silk scaffolds.

Recently, rhBMP-2 delivered via silk fibroin scaffolds in combination with human mesenchymal stem cells was reported, with promising results, in the healing of critical-sized defects of femurs in rats. Compared with other protein-based materials, such as collagen, *silks have distinguishable mechanical properties, presenting slower degradation times and thus allowing adequate time for proper bone remodelling.*

For this reason, silk is a feasible and potential option as a carrier for the controlled delivery of BMPs and, in general, for generating diverse bone tissue-engineering constructs for clinical applications.

Other possible sources of natural polymers for BMP delivery include soy, casein, polyhydroxyalkanoate, polyhydroxybutyrate, corals, carrageenan, gellan gum, agarose and other fibrous proteins, such as keratin and elastin **(Kirker-Head et al, 2007)**[105].

4) Ceramics

Many studies have been dedicated to the understanding of the processes of bone mineralization and it was concluded that ceramic materials, such as hydroxyapatite (HA) and other types of calcium phosphates, can, when implanted, promote the formation of a bone-like mineral surface layer that leads to an increased interface between the materials and the surrounding bone.

Calcium phosphate for tissue engineering of bone includes the use of calcium phosphate layers, films or coatings to promote bone ingrowth, and the use of calcium phosphate fillers to replace fractured or damaged bone. Hydroxyapatite (HA) is a form of calcium phosphate mineral that comprises 70% of bone and can be formulated as a powder, granules, disks or blocks **(Tsuruga et al, 1997)**[126]. The BMP is biomimetically deposited during the formation of the calcium phosphate film that is formed when the material is immersed in a solution of simulated body fluid that mimics the human blood plasma.

Alternatively, bioactive glass (45S5 – Bioglass), a synthetic surface reactive glass that is commonly used as a filler for damaged or fractured bone, may be also used to form biomimetic calcium phosphate-coated scaffolds. The biomimetic layers, similar to bone apatite, may be used in combination with BMPs to guide the attachment and differentiation of bone precursor cells, given that the coatings have been shown to promote osteointegration and osteoinduction.

Promising potential arises from the fact that bioglass is osteoconductive and osteoinductive, stimulating the recruitment and differentiation of osteoblasts, which produce new bone and completely resorb the material.

5) Microparticles and nanoparticles for BMP delivery

The search for efficient, simple and cheap delivery systems for drug targeting has led to great investment in the area of nanoparticles and microparticles for drug delivery. Most common materials for the design of nanodevices to deliver BMPs include synthetic materials, natural polymers and hydroxyapatite-based particles. Both nano-scale (up to 100 nm) and microspheres are reported.

Polylactic acid and polylactic-co-glycolic acid have been used as materials for nanoparticle-based delivery systems for BMPs. PLA was initially studied as a carrier for BMPs in a rat ectopic bone formation model **(Saitoh *et al*, 1994)**[127], showing formation of new bone at 4 weeks after implantation and mature bone after 24 weeks. However, by blending PLA with polyglycolic acid in copolymer polylactic-co-glycolic acid (PLGA), biodegradation is controlled by changing the proportions of each of the two materials, since PLA degrades much more slowly than PGA.

The group concluded that the carrier delivered rhBMP-7 in a time-controlled manner and induced significant bone formation. Diverse natural origin materials were also proposed as carriers at a nano and micro-scale for delivering BMPs.

CHAPTER 09
BMP AND TISSUE REGENERATION

The history of bone morphogenetic proteins began with the observation that demineralized bone matrix (DBM) is able to induce ectopic bone formation in subcutaneous and intramuscular pockets in rodents[1,9]. This bone induction process has been studied extensively[3,4]. Histological and biochemical analysis showed that cartilage appears 5–10 days after implantation of active DBM[24]. This cartilage mineralizes by day 7–14 and is subsequently replaced by bone. After 21 days, haematopoietic bone marrow formation can be observed. These cellular events observed after DBM implantation mimic embryonic bone development and normal fracture repair. As DBM-related bone formation was observed to occur at ectopic sites, it was assumed that *pleuripotent mesenchymal cells are attracted to the site of implantation*. Isolation of the bone-inducing substance revealed that certain proteins were responsible, which were termed bone morphogenetic proteins (BMPs) or osteogenetic proteins (OPs).

The use of *DBM in treating bone defects has proven beneficial* for bone regeneration both in animals and in humans[128-129]. DBM has become widely accepted as a bone-graft substitute in clinical practice, but its bone inductive capacity has been questioned[130-131].

In several studies, *histology revealed that new bone was generated by osteoconduction rather than osteoinduction*[132] – that, bone regeneration occurred by growth of existing host bone on the DBM granules, which acted as a scaffold, rather than by *de novo* differentiation of bone, independent of pre-existing bone.

Lack of inductive properties of DBM may be related to the procedures of production of commercially available DBM, as preservation of osteoinductive activity can be affected by the processing or sterilization procedures. It is also possible that DBM of human origin, which is preferred for use in clinical practice, is less osteoinductive than DBM derived from animals, which is commonly used in animal studies.

Several studies show that *DBM from long-lived species such as baboon and human was not able to induce bone differentiation in short-lived animals such as rats, mice and guinea pigs*[133]. Allogenic intramuscular implantation of *DBM in adult monkeys also failed to induce the formation of bone and produced only strongly delayed bone formation*, 72 days after subcutaneous implantation.

Sampath and Reddi[24] suggested that this limited cross-reactivity was caused by immunogenic factors in crude BMP extracts, which inhibited the bone induction process. Indeed when *BMPs were purified and reconstituted with inactive DBM, bone induction was observed in different species*[134]. Purified human BMP has been used in a number of clinical cases, to repair resistant non-unions and segmental defects of long bones[135-136].

Identification Of Single BMPs And Their Role In Osteoinduction

BMPs belong to the transforming growth factor-β (TGF-β) super-family, which consists of a group of related peptide growth factors. More than 40 related members of this family have been identified, including BMPs, growth and differentiation factors (GDFs), inhibins/ activins, TGF-β's and Mullerian inhibiting substance. Members of the TGF-β superfamily are synthesized as large precursor molecules, and the mature protein is released from a propeptide region by proteolitic cleavage).

BMPs consist of dimers that are interconnected by seven disulphide bonds; this dimineralisation is a prerequisite for bone induction[27]. BMPs are active both as homodimer molecules that consist of two identical chains, and as a heterodimers consisting of two different chains. BMPs have currently been identified[137-138], and they are further divided into subfamilies according to their amino acid sequence similarities.

BMPs 2 and 4 form one subgroup,
BMPs-5–8 form a second subgroup,
a third subgroup contains BMP-3 and GDF-10, a related growth factor.

Members of each subgroup have shown osteoinductivity, with an identical mechanism as observed after ectopic implantation of osteoinductive DBM. BMP-1 is not related to the BMP family. It does not show osteoinductivity[139] and has recently been identified as procollagen-C-proteinase.

In vitro studies of the effects of BMP support the theory that multipotent cells play a role in bone induction *in vivo*. Multipotent cells, either from pre- or postnatal animals or from animal and human bone marrow, showed responsiveness to various BMPs. Newborn rat calvarial cells and rat osteosarcoma cells showed osteogenic differentiation after treatment with recombinant human (rh)OP-1[140]. The fibroblastic cell line, C3H10T1/2, established from an early mouse embryo, showed osteoinductive responses to rhBMP-2. Rat and mouse bone marrow have shown responsiveness to rhBMP-2 by an increase in osteoblastic parameters, human bone marrow has shown an increase in osteoblastic parameters after rhBMP-2 or rhOP-1 treatment. Treatment of primary human bone marrow stromal cells with rhOP-1 resulted in a concentration dependent increase of the osteogenic parameter alkaline phosphatase.

The differentiation stage of multipotent cell populations was found to be an important determinant of the effects of BMP. Whereas myoblasts retained the ability to change their differentiation pathway to express osteoblast parameters, several studies have shown that BMPs do not stimulate mature osteoblasts[141]; moreover, mature fibroblasts could not be induced to express osteogenic parameters after treatment with BMP-2. These results indicate that the *osteogenic influence of BMPs is directed towards immature and multipotent cells. Mature cells seem to loose their responsiveness.*

In healing fractures, which contain many immature cells, expression of native BMPs has been demonstrated, indicating that these proteins have a local regulatory role during fracture repair. As cells derived from non-healing fractures did show an osteogenic response to BMP, it is possible that failure of fracture healing may derive from an insufficient BMP supply.

Few studies have compared the effects of various BMPs directly within one experiment. Mayer and coworkers[142] showed that different BMPs varied in their mitogenic capacity in cultures of periosteal cells and epiphyseal and sternal chondrocytes derived from chick embryos. DNA synthesis increased more after treatment with BMPs 2 and 4 than after BMPs 5 or 6 treatment; the effects of OP-7 were marginal, and BMP- 3 had no effect.

Differences in osteogenic effect have been demonstrated in some studies, but the results are somewhat conflicting. Takuwa and coworkers[139] showed that BMP-2 was able to stimulate alkaline phosphatase activity and collagen synthesis in MC3T3- E1 cells, whereas BMP-3 stimulated collagen synthesis only.

BMP-6 was found to increase the osteoblastic phenotype in secondary rat calvarial cell cultures more than twice as much as BMPs 2 or 4, and BMP 2 was more potent than BMP 4. BMP 6 was a more potent stimulator of bone formation than BMPs 2 and 4 in rat osteoblasts. However, in several bone marrow cell lines, *BMP 6 showed less osteogenic potential than BMPs 2 and 4.*

The identification of BMP receptors and intracellular signal transduction after ligand binding is an area of intensive research that has been reviewed recently[143-145]. Receptors for BMPs are complexes of two different types of membrane-bound serine/threonine kinases: type I BMP receptors, BMPR-1A and BMPR- v1B, and type II receptors. After ligand binding, the type II receptor phosphorylates the type I receptor. The activated type I receptor then phosphorylates a member of the Smad family of intracellular proteins, which are the functional signal transducers of the TGF-β / BMP family[146].

The Smad superfamily can be subdivided into classes I-III. After binding of a BMP to its receptor, Smad 1 and 5 (class I Smads) form heteromeric Smad–Smad complexes with Smad 4 (class II Smad). The complexes regulate molecular transcriptional responses directly. Smads 6 and 7 (class III Smads) are inhibitors of TGF-β / BMP signalling.

Bone: Formation By Induction

Since antiquity, bone has been known to have a remarkable potential for repair and regeneration. Tissue engineering, defined as the science of fabrication of new tissues for replacement and the regeneration of lost or destroyed tissues, has learned and is still learning, the secrets of its principles from bone repair and regeneration, and it is likely that more secrets still remain to be learned from the principles of bone tissue engineering.

The three critical ingredients for optimal tissue engineering are
- *soluble molecular signals,*
- *responding cells with associated cell-surface receptors, and*
- *assembly of the extracellular matrix.*

The accrued knowledge can now be applied not only to bone regeneration, but also to alveolar bone with associated cementum and periodontal ligament regeneration, tissues that are known to be recalcitrant to heal and regenerate.

The complex tissue morphologies of the periodontal tissues are a superb example of design architecture and engineering. The supportive alveolar bone consists of cortical or compact bone and cancellous or trabecular bone. The periodontal ligament system, epitomized by inserting Sharpey's fibers into the cementum, provides a gomphosis that uniquely articulates the tooth to the alveolar bone and permits mechanical function and adaptation to changing mechanical environments and signals additionally modulated by the avascular mineralized root cementum.

There is a direct relationship between differentiation in early development and regeneration in postnatal life. Fracture repair recapitulates events that occur during the normal course of embryonic bone development. The tissue response elicited by heterotopic implantation of demineralized bone matrix is reminiscent of embryonic bone development. Unlike the epiphyseal growth plate, however, where a continuum of cartilage and bone differentiation is observed, in the demineralized matrixinduced bone differentiation, a single cycle of endochondral bone formation is evident.

The sequential developmental cascade includes:
- *Activation and migration of undifferentiated mesenchymal cells by chemotaxis;*
- *Anchoragedependent cell attachment to the matrix via fibronectin,*
- *Mitosis and proliferation of responding mesenchymal cells;*

> *Differentiation of chondroblasts and deposition of cartilage;*
> *Mineralization of the cartilage;*
> *Angiogenesis, vascular invasion and chondrolysis;*
> *Differentiation of osteoblasts and bone matrix deposition; and,*
> *Finally, mineralization of the newly induced bone and differentiation of hemopoietic marrow in the newly formed ossicles.*

The operational reconstitution of the inactive and insoluble collagenous bone matrix with protein extracts after a single step of gel-filtration chromatography restored the biological activity, yielding endochondral bone differentiation by induction after recombining the insoluble with the soluble signals. The dissociative extraction and the operational reconstitution of the matrix components were instrumental to purify BMPs/OPs to homogeneity, yielding amino acid sequences for cloning of the human proteins. The operational econstitution of the soluble and insoluble components of the extracellular matrix of bone pointed to the requirement of an insoluble signal or substratum to deliver the osteogenic activity of the soluble molecular signal. Following increasingly refined purification procedures of the solubilised proteins extracted from demineralized bone matrices, MPs/OPs were isolated and purified in sufficient quantities to provide amino acid sequence information.

Four important technical developments were instrumental for the characterization of the family of the BMPs/OPs:
1) The development of a functional bioassay in the subcutaneous space of the rat to monitor the biological activity of osteogenic proteins[19];
2) Purification schemes utilizing heparin-affinity chromatography[147];
3) The use of electro-endosmotic elution techniques after preparative sodium dodecyl sulfate electrophoresis to achieve final purification to homogeneity;
4) The use of recombinant DNA technologies to clone and express several human BMPs / OPs[26].

Endochondral bone induction is the result of the combinatorial action of BMPs/OPs and the complementary substratum that delivers the osteogenic activity of the soluble molecular signal[26]. After initiation of the first wave of bone differentiation, including the clonal expansion of osteoprogenitor stem cells, the osteogenic cascade is promoted and maintained by a variety of other morphogens of the transforming growth factor-b superfamily, including the transforming growth factor-β isoforms per se.

In the matrix-induced endochondral bone formation, transforming growth factor-β was detected from day 9 onwards after heterotopic subcutaneous implantation in rodents. An increasing concentration correlated with the induction of angiogenesis and the calcification of cartilage. Transforming growth factor-β was found to be compartmentalized in the newly formed and mineralized bone matrix as a mechanism for storage of the latent or processed morphogen.

From Bone Induction To Cementogenesis And Periodontal Ligament Regeneration

More than 40 related proteins with BMP/OP-like sequences and activities have been sequenced and cloned. By default, each protein either purified to homogeneity from natural sources or cloned and expressed by recombinant DNA technology induces endochondral bone formation, by induction, in heterotopic sites of a variety of animal models, including adult primates[148]. *Highly purified naturally derived BMPs/OPs, extracted and purified from baboon and bovine bone matrices, induce complete regeneration of calvarial defects in the adult baboon Papio ursinus*[148].

The endogenous mechanisms of bone repair and regeneration may require the concerted action of several of the BMPs/ OPs present within the natural milieu of the bone matrix. *Complete regeneration may be the result of the sum of a plurality of*

BMP/OP activities, or the result of synergistic interaction amongst the partially purified BMPs/OPs from bone matrices[149]. In addition to bone induction, BMPs/OPs are expressed during early development and organogenesis in Drosophila melanogaster, nematodes and Xenopus laevis, as well as in mammals, indicating that BMPs/OPs and related members play critical roles as soluble mediators of epithelial–mesenchymal interactions and inductive events unrelated to bone induction[149]

In situ hybridization, immune-localization and in vivo studies in mammals, including human primates, have indicated that fruit flies, frogs and fractures share common morphogenetic and inductive mechanisms (i.e. the pleiotropic cascade of activities of BMP/OP gene products). DPP and 60A gene products in the fruit fly D. melanogaster are homologues of human BMPs/OPs, so much so that heterotopic implantation of recombinant hDPP and h60A in heterotopic sites of rodents induce endochondral bone differentiation.

Nature has had a powerful lesson to teach: to initiate the emergence of the skeleton and thus of the vertebrates, Nature has found it easier to use gene products and amino acid sequences already in existence – more than a billion years in the fruit fly D. melanogaster – rather than devise new gene products responsible for the emergence of the skeleton. Specific amino acid variations yielded several homologous morphogenetic proteins, all of which were endowed with the striking prerogative of initiating bone formation by induction culpting the architecture of the skeleton, a unique construct assembling the vertebrate animal[149].

Ultimately, predictable bone regeneration in preclinical and clinical contexts requires information concerning the expression and cross-regulation of gene products of the osteogenic proteins of the transforming growth factor-β superfamily elicited by a single application of a recombinant morphogen[150]. Using the calvarium and the rectus abdominis muscle of adult baboons as a model for tissue induction and morphogenesis, a study investigated the induction of bone morphogenesis by gamma irradiated hOP-1 delivered by gamma-irradiated bovine-insoluble collagenous bone matrix, the hOP-1 osteogenic device, for bone induction in heterotopic and orthotopic sites of the primate P. Ursinus[149]. Tissue induction and morphogenesis were found to be correlated to the expression patterns of OP-1, collagen type IV, BMP-3 and transforming growth factor-β mRNAs, elicited by increasing the dose of single applications of the hOP-1 osteogenic devices (0.0, 0.1, 0.5, and 2.5 mg hOP-1/g of matrix) applied heterotopically in the rectus abdominis muscle and orthotopically in 48 calvarial defects of 12 adult baboons.

Histology and histomorphometry analysis performed on serial undecalcified sections prepared from the specimens harvested on days 15, 30 and 90 showed that the 0.1, 0.5 and 2.5 mg hOP-1 of the hOP-1 osteogenic device induced bone formation, culminating in complete calvarial regeneration by day 90. Expression of type IV collagen mRNA, a marker of angiogenesis, was strongly expressed in both heterotopic and orthotopic tissues.

High expression levels of OP-1 mRNA demonstrated autoinduction of OP-1 mRNAs. Expression levels of BMP-3 mRNA varied from tissues induced in heterotopic vs. orthotopic sites with high expression in rapidly forming heterotopic ossicles together with high expression of type IV collagen mRNA. The temporal and spatial expressions of transforming growth factor-b1 mRNA indicate a specific temporal transcriptional window during which expression of transforming growth factor-β is mandatory for successful and optimal osteogenesis.

The induction of bone by hOP-1 in P. ursinus develops as a mosaic structure with distinct spatial and temporal patterns of gene expression of members of the transforming growth factor-b superfamily that singly, synergistically and synchronously initiate and maintain tissue induction and morphogenesis. The expression of OP-1, type IV collagen, BMP-3 and transforming growth factor-β mRNAs by Northern blot analyses showed a temporal and spatial pattern of expression, indicating progressing stages of osteogenic differentiation during the initiation of bone formation by the hOP-1 osteogenic device. The continuous temporal and spatial high-expression patterns of type IV collagen mRNA indicates the critical role of hOP-1 in the induction of angiogenesis.

Angiogenesis is a prerequisite for osteogenesis; continuous vascularization explains mechanistically the sustained osteogenesis induced by the hOP-1 osteogenic device supported by prominent vascular invasion. The biosynthesis and supramolecular assembly of the perivascular extracellular matrix of invading sprouting capillaries during the initiation of bone formation will ultimately provide the extent of regeneration of the treated calvarial defects and, in addition, will play pivotal physiological roles by sequestering both angiogenic and osteogenic proteins[151].

To sculpt tissue morphogenesis, nature relies on common (yet limited) molecular mechanisms tailored to initiate the emergence of specialized tissues and organs, including the periodontal tissues. Nature's parsimony in sculpting tissue constructs is epitomized by the deployment of a restricted family of molecularly different, but functionally homologous, proteins with minor variations in amino acid motifs within highly conserved C-terminal regions, all endowed with the striking prerogative of initiating endochondral bone formation by induction in addition to specialized pleiotropic functions.

We have learned that signaling networks deployed in both Drosophila and mammalian development, including development of the limbs and the emergence of osteogenesis and thus skeletogenesis, are also deployed in tooth morphogenesis[152] during epithelial–mesenchymal interactions in tooth development[153].

BMPs/OPs are involved in tooth morphogenesis at different stages of development as temporally and spatially connected events[152]. During the later developmental stages of tooth morphogenesis, the induction of cementogenesis, periodontal ligament and alveolar bone differentiation, is regulated by the co-ordinated expression of BMPs/OPs family members[152]. Tissue induction and morphogenesis of the complex tissue morphologies of the periodontal tissues in postnatal life recapitulate embryonic development.

The mosaicism of the expression of gene products during embryonic development is recapitulated postnatally by the exogenous application of highly purified, naturally derived, BMPs/OPs and of single recombinant osteogenic proteins. A systematic analysis of the expression of six different Bmps in tooth morphogenesis has shown that whilst the expression patterns of each Bmp is different, there is co-distribution between specific family members[152-153].

Root morphogenesis is a classical example of epithelial–mesenchymal interactions[152]. In this context, the localization of BMP-3 and OP-1 during morphogenesis of the mouse root (from the developmental stages of mantle dentine deposition) suggests that these proteins play a role during cementogenesis and the assembly of a functionally oriented periodontal ligament fiber system[153]. The localization of BMP-2 in alveolar bone only, and of BMP-3 and OP-1 in all three components of the periodontium, indicates that the morphogenesis of periodontal tissues may involve a composite pattern of co-ordinated expression of different signaling isoforms[153], each endowed with the striking prerogative of initiating bone formation by induction.

The mosaicism of BMP/OP expression during root morphogenesis indicates that optimal therapeutic regeneration and tissue engineering may entail binary combinations of osteogenic gene products based on recapitulation of embryonic development[153].

Structure–Activity Profile And Therapeutic Significance Of Redundancy

BMPs/OPs are involved in inductive events that control pattern formation during morphogenesis in such disparate tissues and organs as the kidney, eye, nervous system, lung, skin, heart and teeth[153-154]. BMPs/OPs induce de novo endochondral bone formation and act as soluble signals of tissue morphogenesis, sculpting the multicellular mineralized structures of the periodontal tissues with functionally oriented periodontal ligament fibers inserted into newly formed cementum.

Amino acid sequence variations in the C-terminal domain confer specialized and pleiotropic activities to each isoform, the molecular basis of the structure–activity profile of each morphogenetic protein. The presence of multiple forms of BMPs/OPs has therapeutic significance, and the choice of a suitable isoform is a formidable challenge for the practicing skeletal reconstructionist and periodontologist alike[31,78]. Amino acid sequence variations in the active C-terminal domain of each morphogenetic protein confer specialized activities to a BMP/OP isoform, and this is the molecular basis that determines the structure–activity profile of single BMPs/OPs[31-78].

This is the biological significance of redundancy and its therapeutic implication rests on developing a structure–activity profile amongst the members of the BMP/OP family (i.e. to study in vivo the morphogenetic impulse of each single and structurally different recombinant hBMP/OP in primates only, in order to identify the pleiotropic activities of different protein isoforms based on specific amino acid sequences)[78].

Periodontal Tissue Regeneration By Naturally Derived And Recombinant Human BMPs / OP's In The Non Human Primate P. Ursinus

To induce the cascade of bone differentiation, the soluble osteogenic molecular signals of the transforming growth factor-β super family must be reconstituted with an insoluble signal or substratum that triggers the bone differentiation cascade[155]. Different BMPs/OPs, and combinations there of, have been implanted in furcation defects of the mandibular first and second molars of adult baboon, P. ursinus, delivered by insoluble collagenous bone matrices as a carrier[78].

Naturally derived BMPs/OPs, purified more than 50,000-fold with respect to the initial crude guanidinium hydrochloride extract of bovine bone matrices, induced cementum, periodontal ligament and alveolar bone regeneration in surgically created class II furcation defects of mandibular molars of P. Ursinus. Osteogenic fractions were prepared by extracting bovine demineralized bone matrices with guanidinium-hydrochloride and were purified greater than 70,000-fold by heparin–Sepharose, hydroxyapatite–Ultrogel and gel-filtration chromatography on Sephacryl S-200.

Importantly, for research experiments in preclinical and clinical contexts, far-reaching experiments by **Sampath & Reddi**[24] have shown homology of mammalian bone inductive proteins, and that bovine BMPs/OPs, in conjunction with the allogeneic baboon collagenous matrix, induce bone differentiation, comparable with that of baboon BMPs/OPs, in extraskeletal sites of the baboon[149].

Undecalcified sections of the treated furcation defects showed the induction of cementogenesis as a yet-to-be-mineralized collagenic material and the synthesis of Sharpey's fibers with foci of mineralization within the newly formed cementoid[149]. Sharpey's fibers were shown to unite the newly formed cementum to the regenerated mineralized alveolar bone surfaced by osteoid seams populated by contiguous osteoblasts. It is noteworthy that *Sharpey's fibers were inserted perpendicularly into the newly formed cementum covered by a thin layer of cementoid*[149].

The source(s) of responding cells that initiate cementogenesis and periodontal ligament regeneration are still not well understood. Recent studies have indicated that the periodontal ligament system contains stem cells that have the potential to regenerate cementum and periodontal ligament in vivo[156]. Exogenous applications of selected BMPs/Ops initiate cementogenesis and regulate the assembly of a functionally oriented periodontal ligament system by transforming specific stem cells, capable of differentiation, towards cementoblasts and osteoblasts[149].

In class II furcation defects of mandibular molars of P. ursinus, relatively low doses of hOP-1 (100 and 500 lg/g of xenogeneic bovine collagenous bone matrix as a carrier) induced preferentially cementogenesis[157], indicating that BMPs/OPs have multiple and pleiotropic functions in vivo that are not limited to endochondral bone formation by induction and that there is a structure–activity profile amongst BMPs/OPs in controlling tissue morphogenesis and regeneration[157]. hOP-1, when in contact with dentine extracellular matrix, is preferentially cementogenic, with limited, if any, alveolar bone induction in short-term experiments in P. ursinus at relatively low doses of the recombinant morphogen[157].

On the other hand, in long-term experiments in P. ursinus, using higher doses of the hOP-1 osteogenic device, regeneration of cementum was observed, with coursing Sharpey's fibers uniting the cementum to the newly induced alveolar bone.

Previous studies in P. ursinus assessed healing on root surfaces that had been surgically exposed and planed[158]. While the regeneration of the connective tissue attachment and alveolar bone seemed to be independent of the character of the root surface if the exposed root had been adequately decontaminated[159], more challenging was the demonstration of cementogenesis and alveolar bone regeneration in periodontally induced furcation defects with root surfaces exposed for a relatively long time to periodontal pathogens. Although nonhuman primates, such as P. ursinus, experience naturally occurring site-specific gingivitis[149], the contention still exists that novel regenerative procedures should be tested in animal models with root surfaces exposed by disease[160].

A pathogenic human strain of Porphyromonas gingivalis was inoculated into the furcations areas of the first and second mandibular molars of four adult P. ursinus, twice a month for 12 months, and chronic periodontitis was induced in all four animals, as assessed by probing periodontal pocket depths, intra-oral radiographs, and microbiological analyses that confirmed the presence of P. Gingivalis[149]. Two months after scaling, root planing and a plaque-control regimen, with clinical resolution of gingivitis, mucoperiosteal flaps were elevated to expose class II furcation defects of the affected mandibular molars filled with granulation tissue[149]. After root planing and debridement, 12 furcation defects were implanted with 0.5 or 2.5 mg of gamma irradiated hOP-1 per gram of xenogeneic bovine insoluble collagenous bone matrix as a carrier[149].

Serial undecalcified sections, prepared 6 months after surgery, showed regeneration of alveolar bone and the induction of cementogenesis, with Sharpey's fibers uniting the regenerated bone to the newly formed cementum. Radiographic analysis showed substantial alveolar bone regeneration, even with the lower-dose hOP-1 osteogenic device. Doses of 2.5 mg of the hOP-1 osteogenic device induce complete regeneration and restitutio ad integrum of the treated furcation defects[149].

The induction of cementogenesis is clearly a critical pleiotropic function of hOP-1 in both primate and canine models. The higher hOP-1 doses tested in periodontally induced furcation defects of P. ursinus might have accounted for the observed histological differences between the longterm and the short-term experiments. Moreover, the longer observation period in P. ursinus, of up to 6 months (compared with the previous short-term experiments), might have also been critical in determining the spatially correct morphogenesis of the periodontal tissues within the periodontally induced furcation defects[149].

Synchronous, but spatially distinct, OP-1 and BMP-2 expression during murine root formation points to specific functions of OP-1 and BMP-2 in periodontal tissue morphogenesis and thus regeneration in postnatal life[149]. The co-localization findings of OP-1 and BMP-2 during tooth morphogenesis[153] has suggested that co administration of OP-1 and BMP-2 in recombinant form would result in synergistic tissue morphogenesis as a recapitulation of memory of developmental events in the embryo[153].

Twelve furcation defects, prepared in the first and second mandibular molars of adult P. ursinus, were used to assess whether qualitative periodontal tissue regeneration could be enhanced and tissue morphogenesis modified by binary applications of hOP-1 and hBMP-2. Doses of recombinant proteins were 100 1g of each protein per gram of insoluble collagenous bone matrix as carrier. Approximately 200 mg of carrier matrix was used per furcation defect.

Undecalcified sections were cut for histological and histomorphomctrical analyses on day 60 after healing. hOP-1-treated-furcation defects showed substantial cementogenesis, with scattered remnants of the collagenous carrier. rhBMP-2 applied singly induced greater amounts of mineralized bone and osteoid when compared to hOP-1 alone (Fig. 6F). Binary applications of hOP-1 and hBMP-2 showed superior cementogenesis, as induced by hOP-1.

Although the majority of animal studies involved the use of hOP-1 and hBMP-2 in a variety of clinical settings and animal models, hBMP-6 has also been investigated in a periodontal fenestration defect model in rodents[161]. *The study indicated that hBMP-6 induced significantly more new cementum formation as opposed to control fenestration defects*[161]. hBMP-12 has also become the focus of attention for periodontal regenerative studies[162]. **Wikesjo et al.** evaluated hBMP-12 for periodontal tissue regeneration, particularly periodontal ligament formation. hBMP-12 and hBMP-2 were implanted on absorbable collagen sponges in periodontal defects and the results were compared after 60 days of healing[162]. *Greater bone regeneration was observed in implants treated with hBMP-2, but ankylosis was noted.*

Defects treated with hBMP-12 showed less bone regeneration, but exhibited a functionally oriented periodontal ligament system inserting into newly formed cementum.

In a tooth replantation study using hBMP-12, **Sorensen et al.** noted that the topical application of hBMP-12 to dentine that had been previously denuded of periodontal ligament, failed to have any effect on re-establishing a new periodontal ligament apparatus[163].

Bone Healing In Animal Studies Using BMP

The osteoinductive properties of rhBMP-2, rhOP-1 and purified BMP-3 have been studied in bone defects in animal models. These studies comprise the grafting of a segmental bone defect that does not heal spontaneously during the lifetime of the animal; such a defect is also called a **critical-size defect**. Complete healing of critical-size defects in rat calvariae was observed after grafting fleeces of bovine bone derived collagen that had been soaked in a rhBMP-2 solution[164]. Calcifying cartilage and remineralization of the collagen carrier were observed after 1 week, which was followed by rapid bone formation.

Yasko and coworkers[165] reported healing of femur defects by rhBMP-2 in rats. In sheep, femoral defects showed new bone formation 1 month after grafting with rhBMP-2 and complete radiographic bone union was observed 3 months after grafting; 1 year after grafting, histology showed the presence of woven and lamellar bone[166].

In dogs, mandibular defects were restored by rhBMP-2 within 3 months. The bone quality as measured by biomechanical strength, degree of mineralization and bone thickness improved significantly during the next 3 months[167]. Complete fusion of vertebrae in experimental spinal fusion in dogs was achieved 3 months after grafting with rhBMP-2[168].

Combination of rhBMP-2 with other carriers such as polymers of poly lactic acid (PLA) or poly glycolic acid (PGA), or a combination of both, have also led to healing of bone defects in rabbits and rats[169,170].

Use of rhOP-1 showed similar results. **Cook and coworkers**[171,172] showed that rhOP-1, linked to a carrier of collagen particles derived from bovine bone, restored critical-sized segmental ulnar defects in rabbits and dogs. Complete radiographic union was observed after 2 months in both species. Histology showed that, after 2 months, lamellar bone had formed, with marrow elements and signs of remodelling. The average torsional strength of the unions was comparable to that of intact bone.

A few studies have demonstrated that purified BMP-3 has osteo-regenerative capacities. Purified bovine BMP-3 on a bone collagen carrier aided healing of femoral defects in rats[173] and purified baboon BMP-3 induced complete regeneration of critical-size calvarial defects in baboons within 3 months.

BMPs were also beneficial in maxillofacial surgery in animal studies. In dental extraction sites and in sinus augmentation in chimpanzees, rhOP-1 aided bone formation[174].

In goat maxillary sinus floor elevations, implantation of rhBMP-2 on a collagen carrier showed increased radio-opacity, histological examination revealing the presence of dense trabeculae and bone marrow, but no cortical bone, 12 weeks after surgery[175]. *These data show that rhBMP-2, rhOP-1 and purified osteogenin are able to repair critical-sized defects in various species within a period of 3 months.*

Human Studies With rhBMP-2 or rhOP-1

The first human pilot studies have been published using rhBMP-2 or rhOP-1 on a collagen carrier for bone reconstruction[176-179]. The results of these studies show a large variation among the responses of individual patients. **Boyne and co-workers**[176] implanted collagen sheets soaked in rhBMP-2 solution in the maxillary sinuses of 12 edentulous or partially edentulous patients with severe atrophy of the maxilla. The subsqent increase in height of the treated maxilla varied between 2.3 and 15.7mm. However, rhBMP-2 grafts were unable to form bone when applied in mandibular ridge augmentation[177]. In tooth extraction pockets, where the graft is surrounded by bone, all grafts were replaced with newly formed bone tissue.

The histological evaluation of the effect of rhOP-1 coupled to a collagen carrier, grafted in the maxillary sinuses of three patients with maxillary atrophy was done. Excellent bone formation was found in one of the three patients, but the two other patients showed little or no bone formation after 6 months. In these two patients, persistent device remnants were found, surrounded by fibrous tissue[178]. **Bulstra and coworkers**[179] used rhOP-1 for grafting of six human fibula osteotomies. Five of the six patients showed bone healing, but one patient did not respond to the rhOP-1-containing graft.

The inconsistent results from these clinical pilot studies suggest that certain factors, which are currently unknown, negatively affect the BMP-dependent bone induction process in humans. For a better performance of BMP-containing bone-graft substitutes, these factors need to be elucidated such as Modulating factors, known from animal studies and *in vitro* experiments, BMP concentration, carrier properties and influence of local and systemic growth factors and hormones.

CHAPTER 10
DOSIMETRY

Although BMPs can induce both intramembranous and endochondral ossification, evidence suggests that BMP-2 stimulates only normal intramembranous ossification within surgically created periodontal defects regardless of the dose. The effects of BMP-2 in mandibles also show that healing follows the developmental pattern of bone formation with the normal processes of remodelling[180].

Increasing the BMP-2 dose in non-human primate mandibular defects increases the width and height of the mandible with the development of new cortical bone and functional integration of new bone with the existing mandible[181].

It is not known why periodontal wound healing appears to bypass an endochondral intermediate regardless of the dose[182]. The development of intramembranous or endochondral ossification may be determined locally by genetically determined spatial factors delivering structural and positional information and tension forces such as loading during occlusal function and by the action of endogenous growth factors.

Dose-related responses to BMPs have also been observed in periodontal regeneration. *Increasing the dose of rhBMP-7 has been shown to increase the amount of regeneration in experimentally-induced furcation defects in beagle dogs.* Although all groups developed increased bone formation compared to controls, bone formation and trabecular structure increased with increasing dose with *only the highest dose significantly increasing formation of new attachment.*

In contrast, various doses of rhBMP-2 in an experimentally-induced periodontitis dog model resulted in only very small and insignificant amounts of new bone and cementum formation compared with controls, regardless of rhBMP-2 concentration.

It is difficult to account for large differences in the regenerative outcome between these 2 studies given that the actions of BMP-2 and BMP-7 are similar and both used collagen carriers.

Comparison of concentrations between the 2 studies is difficult as the actual concentration of rhBMP-7 in its collagen carrier is not clearly stated[182]. However, the data would suggest that the concentration of BMP was greater in the BMP-7 study. Therefore, assuming the 2 BMP proteins have similar actions and that the dose accounted for the different effects on regeneration, it is likely that *a critical minimal dose range is required to increase regeneration beyond control levels.*

A dog study evaluating various doses of rhBMP-2 in experimentally-induced periodontal defects reported no increase in ankylosis compared with controls not treated with the growth factor. However, very little regeneration occurred in these animals, contrary to earlier results using the same model.

The earlier study in which teeth with bony defects were submerged under mucoperiosteal flaps showed significant bony regeneration including new bone formation up to the cemento-enamel junction (CEJ) following a single dose of rhBMP-2. However, the development of ankylosis was associated with the coronal aspects near the CEJ where new bone formation had occurred.

As noted earlier, the results also suggest that the submerged defect model has greater regenerative potential compared with the non-submerged defects despite the application of higher doses of rhBMP-2 in the non-submerged model. Alternatively, the dose may have been too high and it alone prevented regeneration rather than the host dictating the outcome. Nevertheless, the non-submerged study may not be a true evaluation of the potential of BMPs at various doses to initiate ankylosis as limited bone growth was observed in both test and control animals.

In contrast, rhBMP-7 in non- submerged dog defects promoted greater regeneration compared to controls and did not promote ankylosis at any of the concentrations tested[182] In addition, when rhBMP-7 was evaluated in non-submerged defects in baboons it promoted regeneration without ankylosis at several concentrations[182].

Taken together, these studies suggest a number of variables may be important in modulating the effects of BMPs including the animal model, the different responses of BMPs between the submerged and non- submerged defects, dose, and perhaps the BMP used.

CHAPTER 11
RELEASE KINETICS

Although a matrix carrier for BMP-2 is not essential to promote bone formation, there are a number of advantages to an appropriate carrier, including localization and retention of BMP to the site of application thus reducing the loading dose, providing a matrix for mesenchymal cell infiltration, provision of a substrate for cell growth and differentiation, a shape that may help define the resulting new bone, and a degradation rate that does not inhibit bone growth and remodeling resulting in fibrous tissue formation or fibrous encapsulation of the carrier[33].

As BMP has an affinity for type I collagen, it would seem reasonable to use a collagen carrier. However, an increase in new bone formation at a distance from the defect site in a rodent model showed that neither a type I viscous collagen gel nor a collagen sponge was able to contain BMP-2 to the defect site[56]. However, several dog experiments using a collagen sponge with rhBMP-2 have not reported any obvious excess new bone formation beyond the defects[183].

Mucoperiosteal flaps may also serve to restrict BMP dispersal. However, the use of rhBMP-2 in a collagen sponge with an ePTFE barrier membrane has been shown to promote new bone formation coronal to the membrane[184]. This suggested that *diffusion of the rhBMP-2 occurred through the membrane.* These findings have important implications with respect to binding characteristics of BMP to the carrier as well as the capacity of the membranes to bind or filter BMPs and other growth modulating agents. The design of a carrier that utilizes a barrier function as well as retaining BMPs by promoting binding or potentially blocking diffusion has important therapeutic applications in the treatment of periodontal defects.

It has been reported that the half-life of BMP in a collagen sponge was less than 12 hours. This may not provide a sufficient exposure for the cells involved in wound healing, as repair requires a number of weeks in the dog model and even longer in humans[185].

However as noted above, BMPs have a significant effect upon periodontal wound healing and this appears to be influenced by dose and carrier release kinetics. Presumably, the healing process is initiated by rhBMP-2 which sets in motion a cascade of cellular events resulting in differentiation of progenitor cells into phenotypes involved in regeneration.

Although rhBMP-2 initiates stem cells along an osteoprogenitor pathway, *the dose may have to be of sufficient concentration to ensure other growth and differentiation factors do not redirect or retard the desired cells osteogenic potential.*

Understanding when to manipulate a cell's differentiation pathway with the application of single or multiple doses of BMPs or other growth agents at the appropriate concentration is required to optimize these molecules effects in periodontal wound healing.

Therefore, the ability to alter the release kinetics of a carrier has advantages. One way would be to change the degradation rate of the carrier. Additionally, the drug release rate could be controlled chemically by altering the cross-linking pattern of the carrier.

Alternatively, the emission of photons at certain wavelengths or the use of magnetic fields or ultrasound could be used to alter the binding characteristics of the growth factor from its carrier. For example, the release profile of BMP from gelatin can be modified by cross-linking the gelatin with glutaraldehyde.

Release kinetics of BMPs in periodontal and osseous regeneration around dental implants have largely been evaluated in bioabsorbable carrier systems. *The major disadvantage of bioabsorbable carriers is the unpredictability of their breakdown during wound healing.* If the carrier is also to function in maintaing space to allow sufficient proliferation and differentiation of osteogenic precursor cells, then the early resorption of the carrier may lead to premature collapse of the space and limited regeneration.

A recent report of a non-resorbable (polyethyl methacrylate) and tetrahydrofurfuryl methacrylate-(PEM/THFM) based polymer system showed an initial fast release of BMP-2 followed by a phase of slow continuous release[115]. This pattern of release has been previously reported with growth hormone from this polymer. The most surprising thing was that the results indicated that the total amount of BMP-2 released was in the range of 90% of the total amount incorporated[115].

Studies in the laboratory showed that continuously delivered rhBMP-2 from this polymer system during the early stages of wound healing in a rat model of periodontal regeneration produced similar levels of new bone formation compared with a single application delivered in a collagen gel and the polymer alone. The PEM/THFM polymer system can be manipulated to control both the amount and the pattern of release by varying the preparation method, the copolymer ratios, and using different monomers to control hydrophilicity.

These results suggest that this inert carrier system may have potential therapeutic applications in regenerative periodontal procedures as a carrier for rhBMP-2 as well as providing space maintenance by retaining its resilient structure.

CHAPTER 12
IMMUNOGENECITY OF BMP'S

Bone morphogenetic proteins are a family of proteins critically important to embryonic development and postnatal bone healing. The initial BMPs were extracted from bone matrix, which contained not only a mixed collection of inductive factors but also several immunogenic matrix factors[186]. Since the first molecular clones of BMPs were characterized, the advent of biotechnology and recombinant DNA technology have led to the production of large quantities of highly purified BMPs.

Although the preclinical safety and efficacy of purified bovine BMP extract had been previously investigated, it is these rh- BMPs that are now being evaluated clinically for use in spinal fusion[187]. *Although recombinant human proteins have proven to be generally less immunogenic than those purified from animal tissues, most of them have been shown to induce antibodies*[188].

The number of preclinical and clinical studies on the use of rhBMPs and the patients receiving rhBMPs are increasing rapidly, but there have only been a few anecdotal reports on the formation of antibodies. The exact incidence and clinical significance of the reported antibodies have not been clearly demonstrated.

Bone morphogenetic proteins have some characteristic features that distinguish them from other therapeutic proteins regarding imunogenicity. Whereas most therapeutic proteins are used to correct an acquired or genetic deficiency caused by the absence or poor expression of a native protein[188], rhBMPs were developed to enhance spinal fusion and fracture healing. That is, BMPs are administered locally to address local challenges in bone regeneration and repair, unlike most therapeutic proteins that are administered systemically.

The route of administration could be an important factor influencing the incidence of antibody induction, as it is accepted that the subcutaneous and intramuscular administration of proteins may be more immunogenic than intravenous, oral, or aerosolized delivery[189]. Bone morphogenetic proteins are proteins secreted as soluble factors that have autocrine and paracrine effects.

Therapeutic application of BMPs does not appear to cause any systemic toxic effects[190]. This feature may be due to the presence of a highly complex autoregulatory system that blocks BMP action at various levels, and the rapid binding of the active BMP molecule to extracellular factors that modulate BMP activity.7

Furthermore, some animal studies suggest that rhBMP-2 is so quickly and extensively cleared from the circulation that the systemic presence is negligible[190]. A recent publication on rabbit lumbar fusion also demonstrated low systemic exposure to implanted OP-1. Because antibody formation is in part related to both the amount of antigen used and the duration of exposure, proteins that are rapidly eliminated from the systemic circulation are less apt to promote immune responses than those with longer half-lives[191].

Hypersensitivity responses may not pose a significant concern in the application of BMPs because they occur infrequently with proteins of human and recombinant origin, particularly in patients with a fully functional endogenous protein counterpart.

As previously described, BMPs are not used to replace deficient proteins but to enhance bone regeneration through more intensive recruitment of cells with osteogenic potential. Thus it is *unlikely that BMPs would appear as foreign proteins to the patient's immune system*. However, repeat dosing of BMPs has not been recommended in patients in whom antibodies are detected because of the potential of developing these strong immune reactions[190].

The mechanism underlying the induction of antibodies against recombinant human proteins involves a "breach" of immune tolerance for the endogenous protein, whereas antibody responses to nonhuman proteins of plant or bacterial origin is based on the classic reaction to foreign material[189].

How the immune tolerance to self-antigens is broken is not completely understood, but one established way to break tolerance is through the repetitive presentation of self-antigens. Although the repeated dosing of other recombinant human proteins such as insulin and growth hormone has not compromised their therapeutic activity, further studies of the clinical consequences of repeated exposure to rhBMPs should be performed.

Carreon et al.[192] have recently demonstrated that multiple exposures to rhBMP-2 did not result in clinically detectable allergic reactions, although assays for antibody responses were not performed. As noted by these authors, complications of neck swelling, dysphagia, and bone resorption after the administration of rhBMP-2 have recently been reported.

However, these complications do not appear to be related to the immune responses, but instead are problems related to high dosage and a direct inflammatory response. The clinical significance of the immune response to exogenously administered rhBMPs remains unclear, and even the exact incidence of non-neutralizing and neutralizing antibody formation against rhBMP-2 and OP-1 has not yet been elucidated.

However, based on the large and growing body of literature from clinical studies involving BMP utilization, it is unlikely that antibodies, if present, provoke life-threatening problems in the manner of pure red cell aplasia caused by the cross-reactivity of antibodies to endogenous erythropoietin. One potential exception could be during pregnancy, in which antibodies to rhBMP could cross the placenta and potentially cause devastating effects in the developing fetus.

In a preclinical study, *rhBMP-2 has been shown to elicit antibodies capable of crossing the placenta*. Because the influence of maternal antibody formation against rhBMP-2 or OP-1 on human fetal development is unknown, the use of BMPs is contraindicated in women with childbearing potential[190]. Preclinical reproductive toxicology studies have been performed in which pregnant female rabbits were hyperimmunized with recombinant OP-1; these rabbits gave birth to normal litters with no observed defects.

There have been several clinical trials of rhBMPs reporting the results of immunogenicity testing, most of which have demonstrated low antibody formation rates. Antibody production was transient and did not appear to affect the incidence of adverse events, fusion rates, or other clinical outcomes.

CHAPTER 13
FUTURE TRENDS & CHALLENGES

In the Western world, an estimated 5–10% of all bone fractures show deficient healing, leading to delayed union or non-union, causing significant morbidity and psychological stress to the patients and bringing elevated costs to society **(Westerhuis et al, 2005)**[193]. Fortunately, the current advances in bone tissue engineering have led researchers to find new strategies and devices with the use of BMPs for accelerating the healing of bone tissues in the orthopaedic field. In fact, by the end of 2007, early 1 million patients worldwide were projected to have been treated with BMPs for diverse bone-related problems and diseases.

The clinical uses of BMPs include spinal fusion, treatment of long bone defects and non-unions, dental and periodontal tissue engineering, craniofacial defects and diseases, fracture repair, the improvement of osteointegration with metallic implants, musculo-skeletal reconstructive surgery and tendon and ligament reconstruction.

There are currently two main collagen-based products containing BMP-2 or BMP-7 that were approved by the FDA in recent years for human clinical use: **Infuse**™ **Bone Graft** (Medtronik, US Wyeth, UK), containing rhBMP-2, and **Osigraft**™ (Stryker Biotech), containing rhBMP-7, known by the designation of OP-1 (osteogenic protein-1).

BMP-2 Infuse™ **bone graft** was approved for certain interbody fusion procedures in 2002, for open tibial fractures in 2004, and for alveolar ridge and sinus augmentations in 2007 **(McKay et al, 2007)**[194].

BMP-7 Osigraft™ was approved for long bone fractures and as an alternative to autografts in patients requiring posterolateral lumbar spinal fusion. There has been also an increasing number of trials that provide supporting evidence for the use of rhBMP-7/OP-1 in the treatment of open tibial fractures, distal tibial fractures, tibial non-unions, scaphoid non-unions and atrophic long bone non-unions **(White et al, 2007)**[195].

Bone repair and regeneration with BMPs are ushering in a new era. The past 10 years have seen practical demonstration of bone repair in a series of animal studies and subsequently in clinical trials. The expected value of BMPs in the treatment of bone defects, spinal fusion applications and other types of related applications is enormous. Extensive research in preclinical models has led to the approval of restricted use for human trials.

However, despite the significant evidence of potential for bone healing demonstrated in animal models, future clinical investigations will be needed to better define variables such as dose, scaffold and route of administration. The impressive results of animal models are difficult to replicate in humans. It is unclear why these differences occur.

Some insight is provided by the clear species-specific dose response, ranging from 25 µg/ml in rodents to 50 µg/ml in dogs, 100 µg/ml in non-human primates and 800 µg/ml in humans **(Luginbuehl et al, 2004)**[196]. The recruitment of bone precursor cells and bone turnover may occur differently in rodents, small animals and large mammals.

Likewise, the dosing may not yet be optimal. In fact, the concentrations of BMP in use are supraphysiological and a million times higher (milligrams in assays as compared to the nanogram range *in vivo*). BMP inhibitors such as noggin or sclerotin, which are upregulated by BMP presence, may be interfering and providing a negative feedback effect on the bodily healing mechanisms **(Westerhuis et al, 2005)**[193].

Understanding the regulation between BMPs and BMP-inhibitors might be a key issue. Moreover, different fractures may require different dosages. Critical issues to consider include the potential risk of BMPs inducing heterotopic bone formation, especially when implanted adjacent to neural tissues, and the serious issue of reported antibody formation, noted in up to 38% of patients in some trials with BMPs.

Clearly, the use of BMPs in orthopaedics is still in its early days, but the latest trials in humans suggest that an exciting and promising future will unfold in the development of novel tissue-engineering products for a wide range of clinical situations, with the use of BMPs.

To date, clinical trials have focused mostly on rhBMP-2 and -7 and with the use of collagen as delivery materials. However, given the intricate network of molecules interplaying during bone regeneration, it is possible that a 'cocktail' of different BMPs with simultaneous or sequential release would be the most desirable approach to clinical uses, instead of a single stimulus or molecule **(Hadjiargyrou *et al*, 2002)**[197].

Nevertheless, in the near future, the emergent advances with recombinant production of BMPs **(Klosch *et al*, 2005; Schmoekel *et al*, 2005; Bessa *et al*, 2007)**[198-200] will aid researchers in obtaining larger amounts of bioactive rhBMPs which could be used for tissue-engineering research and the development of novel products.

With the excitement over the potential of other natural origin polymers as novel delivery systems for BMPs, there is little doubt that these will also find relevant places in regenerative medicine of bone and traumatology, and may be soon approaching clinical trials in humans. Diverse natural-origin polymers have shown promising success for bone tissue engineering, such as fibrin, hyaluronic acid, chitosan, silk fibroin and starch-based composites.

The recent advances in biomaterials science will certainly boost the number of tissue-engineering approaches for the healing of bone with the use of BMPs. Novel strategies will possibly involve the specific targeting of BMPs, in injectable systems and stimulus-responsive hydrogels, the use of nano-scale patterning or encapsulated particles, or with the use of molecules combined with the BMP, mimicking the extracellular matrix, all of which allow restricted and site-specific delivery of these growth factors.

Additionally, the design of 3D specific-architecture scaffolds by methods such as rapid prototyping or the design of bilayered scaffolds surely ensures that the carrier for delivering the BMP will closely mimic the bone structure. Guided tissue-engineering delivery systems, which would deliver not only BMPs but also angiogenic factors, would, for instance, prompt the recruitment and distribution of blood vessel precursor cells, which is necessary for the formation of mature bone.

Finally, the use of Ca-P cements and biomimetic coatings is a very promising approach, since it furthers mimics the bone mineral make-up and aids in retaining the BMP and improving tissue–material integration. The expanding variety of options for biomedical use of BMPs gives the promise that the future of clinical regenerative medicine. and that of BMPs, particularly for bone applications, will be certainly be a bright one in the coming decades for millions of people.

LONG TERM CONCERNS WITH BMP

There are several long-term concerns about the use of recombinantly manufactured BMPs in humans. The effects of high doses of BMP on a developing embryo are unknown. Therefore, at this time its use during pregnancy is not advised. Although it is a human protein, there is a risk of developing an immune reaction to the protein. This risk increases if BMP is administered more than once such as in cases of repeated fusion. The magnitude of this risk remains unknown.

Development of an osteogenic sarcoma is possible, although experimental dose escalation studies in animal models have not induced neoplasm. It is of some concern that spontaneously evolving osteosarcomas contain high levels of BMPs.

Uncontrollable bone growth in the vicinity of the neural structures, especially nerve roots and cauda equina, is a potential problem. This can only be solved using efficient carriers that bind the protein tightly, preventing BMP release during of protein axial loading.

SUMMARY & CONCLUSION

Bone Morphogenetic proteins include a large number of proteins belonging to the TGF – β super family, which are characterised by their ability to induce bone and cartilage formation. Since the isolation and purification of Bone Morphogenetic proteins by recombinant technology, the effects of single Bone Morphogenetic proteins can now be evaluated in animal models.

Subcutaneous placement of a single recombinant Bone Morphogenetic proteins, such as recombitant human (rh) Bone Morphogenetic proteins – 2, in a rat ectopic assay shows recruitment of undifferentiated mesenchymal cells, cartilage formation, followed by replacement with bone, formation of its own bone marrow and physiological bone remodelling.

The therapeutic use of Bone Morphogenetic proteins in the treatment of periodontal disease (destruction of tooth ligaments, surrounding bone and cementum) has attracted considerable interest due to their potent ability to stimulate intramembranous bone formation without an endochondral intermediate. Their predictability in stimulating new bone may provide an alternative that has greater osteogenic potential than autogenous bone , other bone factors and bone substitutes.

The biological processes and the potential role of growth factors involved in promoting regeneration are complicated by the involvement of the different cell types each with their different frowth rates and responses to various growth stimulus.

The major cell types involved in periodontal regeneration includes osteoblasts, cementoblasts and fibroblasts. Here, the formation of new mineralised layers on the tooth and bone surfaces by cementoblasts and osteoblasts respectively are a prerequiste before periodontal ligament formation and attachments by fibroblasts can occur. In this regard, Bone Morphogenetic Proteins are likely candidates to stimulate periodontal regeneration because of their ability not only to promote osteogenesis but also to stimulate cementogenesis (new cementum formation).

However, understanding when to manipulate each of the various cells differentiation pathway with the application of the single or multiple doses of Bone Morphogenetic Proteins at the appropriate concentration is dependent upon a suitable delivery system that can be modified in order to optimize its effect during periodontal wound healing.

Furthermore, treatment of intrabony periodontal defects with Bone Morphogenetic Proteins are likely to not only require appropriate temporal release of the agent, but also adaptation of a carrier that is robust enough to maintain its integrity around the coronal aspect of the root in order to provide space maintenence and support the muco-periosteal flap.

APPENDIX - I

ABBREVIATIONS

- AMH : Anti-mullerian hormone
- ALP : Alkaline Phosphatase
- BAMBI : BMP and Activin membrane bound inhibitor
- BMP : Bone Morphogenetic Proteins
- BMPR : Bone Morphogenetic Protein receptor
- Ca : Calcium
- CDMP : Cartilage-derived morphogenetic protein
- CEJ : Cemento Enamel Junction
- DBM : Demineralised Bone Matrix
- DNA : Deoxyribo-nucleic acid
- Dpp : Drosophila protein
- EDTA : Ethylene diamine tetra acetic acid
- ePTFE : expanded Poly Tetra Fluoro Ethylene
- Fe : Iron
- FCM : Fibrous Collagen Membrane
- FDA : Food And Drug Administration
- FOP : Fibroplasias ossificans progressive
- FGF : Fibroblast growth factor
- GDF : Growth differentiation factor
- HA : Hydroxyapatite
- HCl : Hydro Chloric acid
- HGS : Hepatocyte growth factor regulating substrate
- hBMP : Human Bone Morphogenetic Protein
- IGF : Insulin like growth factor
- mRNA : Messenger Ribo nucleic acid
- MIS : Mullerian inhibiting substances

- NBV : New Bone Volume
- Nacl : Sodium Chloride
- OP : Osteogenic Protein
- PEG : Polyethythlene Glycol
- PEM : Poly Ethyl Methacrylate
- PGA : Polyglycolic acid
- PLA : Polylactic acid
- PLGA : Polylactic – co – glycolic acid
- PDGF : Platelet derived growth factor
- rhBMP : recombitant human Bone Morphogenetic Protein
- SARA : SMAD Anchor For Receptor Activation
- se : Short ear
- TF : Transcription factors
- TGF–β : Transforming growth factor beta
- TGFBR : Transforming growth factor beta receptor
- THFM : Tetra Hydro Furfuryl Methacrylate
- VEGF : Vascular endothelial growth factor
- Vgr : Vegetal related

REFERENCES

1) **Urist MR**. Bone: Formation by auto-induction. *Science.* 1965: 150: 893-899.
2) **Martinovic S, Simic P, Borovecki F, Vukicevic S**. Biology of Bone Morphogenetic Proteins. Regeneration of bone and beyond. *Birkhauser, Basel*: 2004: 45-73.
3) **Reddi AH**. Role of morphogenetic proteins in skeletal tissue engineering and regeneration. *Nat Biotechnol.* 1998: 16: 247–252.
4) **Reddi AH.** 2005; BMPs: from Bone Morphogenetic Proteins to Body Morphogenetic Proteins. *Cytokine Growth Factor Rev.* 2005: 16: 249–250.
5) **Pecina M, Vukicevic S**. Biological aspects of bone, cartilage and tendon regeneration. *Int Orthop*: 2007: 31: 719-720.
6) **Urist MR, Dowell**. Inductive substraction for osteogenesis in pellets of particulate bone matrix. *Clin Orthop & related research.* 1968: 61: 61-78.
7) **Urist MR, Silverman BE, Btiring K, Dubuc FL, Rosenberg JM**. The bone induction principle. *Clinical Orthopaedics and Related Research.* 1967: 53: 243- 283.
8) **Urist MR.** The search for and the discovery of bone morphogenetic protein (BMP). In: *Bone Grafts. Derivatives and Substitutes,* (eds): 315-362. London: Butterworth Heinemann: 1994.
9) **Van de Putte KA, Urist MR**. Experimental mineralization of collagen sponge and decalcified bone. *Clinical Orthopaedics and related research*.1965:40:48-56.
10) **Van de Putte KA, Urist MR**. Osteogenesis in the interior of intramuscular implants of decalcified bone matrix. *Clinical Orthopaedies and Related Research* 1966: 43: 257-270.
11) **Levander G.** A study of bone regeneration. *Surgery, Gynecology and Obstetrics.* 1938: 61: 705-714.
12) **Lacroix P.** Recent investigations on the growth of bone. *Nature* 1945: 156:

576.

13) **Heinen JH, Dabbs GH, Mason HA.** The experimental production of ectopic cartilage and bone in the muscles of rabbits. *The Journal of Bone and Joint Surgery.* 1949: 31A: 765-775.

14) **Young MH.** The repair of experimental defects in rabbit skulls. *The Journal of Bone and Joint Surgery.* 1964: 46B: 329-335.

15) **Urist MR, Strates BS.** Bone Morphogenetic Protein. *Journal of Dental Research.* 1971: suppl. 6: 50: 1392-1406.

16) **Urist MR, Dowell TA, Hay RH, Strates BS.** Inductive substrates for bone Formation. *Clinical Orthopaedics and Related Research.* 1968: 59: 59-96.

17) **Urist MR, Iwata H, Strates BS.** Bone morphogenetic protein and proteinase in the guinea pig. *Clinical Orthopaedics and Related Research.* 1972: 85: 275-290.

18) **Syftestad G, Urist MR.** Degradation of bone matrix morphogenetic activity by pulverization. *Clinical Orthopaedics and Related Research.* 1979: 141: 281-286.

19) **Reddi AH, Huggms CB.** Influence of geometry of transplanted tooth and bone on transformation of fibroblasts. *Proceedings of the Society for Experimental Biology and Medicine.* 1973: 143: 634-637.

20) **Urist MR, Granstein R, Nogami H, Svenson L, Murphy R.** Transmembrane bone morphogenesis across multiple - walled diffusion chambers. *Archives of Surgery.* 1977: 112: 612-619.

21) **Urist MR et al.** A bovine low molecular weight bone morphogenetic protein -BMP fraction. *Clinical Orthopaedics and Related Research.* 1982: 162: 219-231.

22) **Urist MR, DeLange RJ, Finerman GAM.** Bone cell differentiation and growth factors. *Science.* 1983: 220: 680-686.

23) **Urist MR et al.** Purification of bovine bone morphogenetic protein by hydroxyapatite chromatography. *Proceedings of the National Academy of Sciences USA.* 1984: 81: 371-375.
24) **Sampath TK, Reddi AH.** Dissociative extraction and reconstitution of extracellular matrix components involved in local bone differentiation. *Proceedings of the National Academy of Sciences USA.* 1981: 78: 7599-7603.
25) **Wang EA et al.** Purification and characterization of other distinct bone-inducing factors. *Proceedings of ihe National Academy of Sciences USA.* 1988: 85: 9484-9488.
26) **Wozney JM et al.** Novel regulators of bone formation: molecular clones and activities. *Science.* 1988: 242: 1528-1534.
27) **Wozney JM.** Bone morphogenetic proteins. *Progress in Growth Factor Research.* 1989: 1: 267-280.
28) **Wozney JM, Rosen V, Byrne M, Celeste AJ, Moutsatsos I, Wang EA.** Growth factors influencing bone development. *Journal of Celt Science,* 1990 Suppl 13: 149-156.
29) **Celeste AJ, lannazzi JA, Taylor RC, Hewick RM, Rosen V, Wang EA, Wozney JM.** Identification of transforming growth factor β family members present in bone-inductive protein purified from bovine bone. *Proceedings of the National Academv of Sciences* USA. 1990: 87: 9843-9847.
30) **Wozney JM.** Molecular biology of the bone morphogenetic proteins. In *Bone Grafts.Derivatives and Substitutes,* (eds.): pp. 397-413. London: Butterworth Heinemann. (1994)
31) **Ripamonti U, Reddi AH.** Periodontal regeneration: potential role of bone morphogenetic proteins. *Journal of Periodontal Research.* 1994: 29: 225-235.
32) **Massague J.** The transforming growth factor-β family. *Annual Review of Cell Biology.* 1995: 6: 597- 641.
33) **Wozney JM.** The potential role of bone morphogenetic proteins in periodontal reconstruction. *Journal of Periodontology.* 1995: 66: 506-510.

34) **Song JJ, Celeste AJ, Kong FM, Jirtie RL, Rosen V, Thies RS.** Bone morphogenetic protein-9 binds to liver cells and stimulates proliferation. *Endocrinology.* 1995: 136: 4293-4297.

35) **Thompson NL, Flanders KC, Smith JM, Ellingsworth LR, Roberts AB, Sporn MB.** Expression of transforming growth factor- SI in specific cells and tissues of adult and neonatal mice. *Journal of Cell Biology.* 1989: 108: 661-669.

36) **Joyce ME, Roberts AB, Sporn MB, Bolander ME.** Transforming growth factor-β and the initiation of chondrogenesis and osteogenesis in the rat femur. *Journal of Cell Biology.* 1990: 2195-2207.

37) **Burt DW.** Evolutionary grouping of the transforming growth factor-β superfamily. *Biochemical and Biophysical Research Communications.* 1992: 184: 590-595.

38) **Gelbart WM.** The *decapentaptegic* gene: a TGF-β (homologue controling pattern formation in *Drosophila). Development.* 1989: suppl. 1: 65-74.

39) **Lyons K et al.** *Vgr1-* a mammalian gene related to *Xenopus Vgr-1* is a member of the transforming growth factor β Gene super family. *Proceedings of the National Academy of Sciences USA.* 1989: 86: 4554-4558.

40) **Wozney JM.** The bone morphogenetic protein family and osteogenesis. *Molecular Reproduction and Development.* 1992: 32: 160-167.

41) **Storm EE, Huynh TV, Copeland NG, Jenkins NA, Kingsley DM, Lee S.** Limb alterations in *brachypodism* mice due to mutations in a new member of the TGF/β superfamily. *Nature.* 1994: 368: 639-643.

42) **Luyten FP et al.** Purification and partial amino acid sequence of osteogenin – A protein initiating bone differentiation. *Journal of Biological Chemistry.* 1989: 264: 13377-13380.

43) **Reddi AH.** Regulation of cartilage and bone differentiation by bone morphogenetic proteins. *Current Opinion in Cell Biology.* 1992: 4: 850-855.

44) **Kingsley DM, Bland AE, Grubber JM, Marker PC, Russell LB, Copeland NG, Jenkins NA.** The mouse *short ear* skeletal morphogenesis locus is associated with defects in a bone morphogenetic member of the TGF-β superfamily. *Cell.* 1992: 71: 399-410.
45) **Kingsley DM.** What do BMPs do in mammals? Clues from the mouse short-ear mutation. *Trends in Genetics.* 1994: 10: 16-21.
46) **Tabas JA et al.** Bone morphogenetic protein: Chromosomal localization of human genes for BMP 1, BMP 2 and BMP 3. *Genomics.* 1991: 9: 283-289.
47) **Hahn GV, Cohen RB, Wozney JM, Levitz CL, Shore EM, Zaslof MA, Kaplan FS.** A bone morphogenetic protein subfamily: Chromosomal localization of human genes for BMP 5, BMP 6. and BMP 7. *Genomics.* 1992: 14: 759-762.
48) **Tabas JA et al.** Chromosomal assignment of the human gene for bone morphogenetic protein 4. *Clinical Orthopaedics and Related Research.* 1993: 293: 310-316.
49) **Barton DE, Yang-Feng TL, Mason AJ, Seeburg PH, Francke U.** Mapping of genes for inhibiting subunit αβA. and βB on human and mouse chromosomes and studies of *jsd* mice. *Genomics.* 1989: 5: 91-99.
50) **Padgett RW, Wozney JM, Gelbart WM.** Human BMP sequences can confer normal dorsal-ventral patterning in the *Drosophila* embryo. *Proceedings of the National Academy of Sciences USA.* 1993: 90: 2905-2909.
51) **Sampath TK, Rashka KE, Doctor JS, Tucker RF, Hoffman FM.** *Drosophila* transforming growth factor β superfamily proteins induce endochondral bone formation in mammals. *Proceedings of the National Academy of Sciences USA.* 1993: 90: 6004-6008.
52) **Hogan BLM, Blessing M, Winnier GE, Suzuki N, Jones CM.** Growth factors in development: the role of TGF-β related polypeptide signalling molecules in embryogenesis. *Development.* 1994: suppl: 53-60.

53) **Lyons KM, Pelton RW, Hogan BLM.** Organogenesis and pattern formation in the mouse: RNA distribution patterns suggest a role for Bone Morphogenetic Protein-2A (BMP-2A). *Development.* 1990: 109: 833 - 844.

54) **Ebara S, Nakayama K.** Mechanism for the action of bone morphogenetic proteins and regulation of their activity. *Spine.* 2002: Aug 15: 27: (16 Suppl 1) :S10-5.

55) **Weiss RE, Reddi AH**: Synthesis and localisation of fibronectin during collagenous matrix mesenchymal cell interaction and differentiation of cartilage and bone in vivo. *Proc Nat Acad Sci USA.* 1980: 77: 2074 – 2078.

56) **King GN, King N, Hughes FJ.** Effect of two delivery systems for recombinant human bone morphogenetic protein -2 on periodontal regeneration in vivo. *J Periodont Res.* 1998: 33: 226 – 236.

57) **Reddi AH.** Cell biology and biochemistry of endochondral bone development. *Cell Rel Res.* 1981: 1: 209-226.

58) **Alberts B, Alexander J, Julian L, Martin R, Keith R, Peter W.** Molecular Biology of the Cell. New York, NY: Garland Science. 2002.

59) **Munir S, Xu G, Wu Y, Yang B, Lala PK, Peng C.** Nodal and ALK7 inhibit proliferation and induce apoptosis in human trophoblast cells. *J Biol. chem.* 2004: 279: (30): 31277–31286.

60) **Wrana JL, Attisano L, Carcamo J et al.** TGF beta signals through a heteromeric protein kinase receptor complex. *Cell.* 1992: 71 (6): 1003 -1014.

61) **Runyan CE, Schnaper HW, Poncelet AC.** The role of internalization in transforming growth factor β1-induced Smad2 association with Smad anchor for receptor activation (SARA) and Smad2-dependent signalling in human mesenchymal cells. *J. Biol. Chem.* 2005: 280 (9): 8300–8308.

62) **Moustakas A.** Smad signalling network. *J. Cell. Sci.* 2002: 115: 3355–3356.

63) **Souchelnytskyi S, Ronnstrand L, Heldin CH, Dijke P.** Phosphorylation of Smad signaling proteins by receptor serine/threonine kinases. *Methods Mol. Biol.* 2001: 124: 107–20.

64) **Massague J, Chen YG.** Controlling TGF-beta signaling. *Genes Dev.* 2000: 14 (6): 627–44.

65) **Blobe GC, Liu X, Fang SJ, How T, Lodish HF.** A novel mechanism for regulating transforming growth factor beta (TGF-beta) signaling. Functional modulation of type III TGF-beta receptor expression through interaction with the PDZ domain protein, GIPC. *J. Biol. Chem.* 2001: 276 (43): 39608–39617.

66) **Itoh F, Asao H, Sugamura K, Heldin CH, ten Dijke P, Itoh S.** Promoting bone morphogenetic protein signaling through negative regulation of inhibitory Smads. *Embo J.* 2001: 20(15): 4132–4142.

67) **Seeherman H, Wozney JM.** Delivery of bone morphogenetic proteins for orthopaedic tissue regeneration.*Cytokine Growth Factor Rev.* 2005: 16: 329–345.

68) **Bessa PC, Casal M, Reis RL.** Bone morphogenetic proteins in tissue engineering: the road from laboratory to clinic, part II (BMP delivery). *J Tissue Eng Regen Med* 2008: 2: 81–96.

69) **Groeneveld HHJ, Van den Bergh JPA, Holzmann P, Ten Bruggenkate CM, Tuinzing DB & Burger EH**. Mineralization processes in demineralized bone matrix grafts in sinus floor elevations. *Journal of Biomedical Materials and Research.* 1999: 48: 393–402.

70) **Nimb L, Jensen JS, Gotfredsen K**. Interface mechanics and histomorphometric analysis of hydroxyapatite-coated and porous glass-ccramic implants in canine bone. *Journal of Biomedical Materials Research.* 1995: 29: 1477–1482.

71) **Gao TJ, Lindholm TS, Kommonen B, Ragni P, Paronzini A & Lindholm TC.** Microscopic evaluation of bone–implant contact between hydroxyapatite, bioactive glass and tricalcium phosphate implanted in sheep di-physeal defects. *Biomaterials.* 1995: 16: 1175–1179.

72) **Verheyen CC, Wijn JR, Blitterswijk CA, Groot K, Rozing PM.** Hydroxylapatite/(poly)L-lactide composites: an animal study on push-out

strengths and interface histology. *Journal of Biomedical Materials Research.* 1993: 27: 433–444.

73) **Shi S, Kirk M, Kahn AJ.** The role of type I collagen in the regulation of the osteoblast phenotype. *J Bone and Mineral Res.* 1996: 11: 1139–1145.

74) **Muthukumaran N, Reddi AH.** Dose-dependence of and threshold for optimal bone induction by collagenous bone matrix and osteogenin-enriched fraction. *Collagen Related Research.* 1988: 8: 433–441.

75) **Otto TE, Klein CPAT, Patka P, Vries R.** Intramedullary bone formation after polylactic acid wire implantation. *Journal of Materials Science: Materials in Medicine.* 1994: 5: 407–410.

76) **Otto TE, Klein-Nulend J, Patka P, Burger EH & Haarman HJ.** Effect of (poly)-L-lactic acid on the proliferation and differentiation of primary bone cells *in vitro*. *Journal of Biomedical Materials Research.* 1996: 32: 513–518.

77) **Hollinger JO.** Preliminary report on the osteogenic potential of a biodegradable copolymer of polylactide (PLA) and polyglycolide (PGA). *Journal of Biomedical Materials Research.* 1983: 17: 71–82.

78) **Ripamonti U.** Osteoinduction in porous hydroxyapatite implanted in heterotopic sites of different animal models. *Biomaterials.* 1996: 17: 31–35.

79) **DeLustro F, Dasch J, Keefe J, Ellingsworth L.** Immune responses to allogeneic and xenogeneic implants of collagen and collagen derivatives. *Clinical Orthopaedics and Related Research.* 1990: 260: 263–279.

80) **Tomford WW.** Transmission of disease through transplantation of musculoskeletal allografts. *Journal of Bone and Joint Surgery, American Volume.* 1995: **77:** 1742–1754.

81) **Nimb L, Jensen JS, Gotfredsen K.** Interface mechanics and histomorphometric analysis of hydroxyapatite-coated and porous glass-ceramic implants in canine bone. *Journal of Biomedical Materials Research.* 1995: 29: 1477–1482.

82) **Matsuda M, Kita S, Takekawa M, Ohtsubo, Tsuyama K.** Scanning electron and light microscopic observations on the healing process after sintered bone implantation in rats. *Histology and Histopathology.* 1995: 10: 673–679.

83) **Zegzula HD, Buck DC, Brekke J, Wozney JM, Hollinger JO.** Bone formation with use of rhBMP-2 (recombinant human bone morphogenetic protein-2). *Journal of Bone and Joint Surgery, American Volume.* 1997: 79: 1778–1790.

84) **Baron R & Saffar JL.** Bone remodeling during experimental periodontal disease in the golden hamster: a quantitative study. *Journal of Periodontal Research.* 1978: 13: 309–315.

85) **Ijiri S, Nakamura T, Fujisawa Y, Hazama M, Komatsudani S.** Ectopic bone induction in porous apatite–wollastonite-containing glass ceramic combined with bone morphogenetic protein. *Journal of Biomedical Materials Research.* 1997: 35: 421–432.

86) **Oda S, Kinoshita A, Higuchi T, Shizuya T, Ishikawa I.** Ectopic bone formation by biphasic calcium phosphate (BCP) combined with recombinant human bone morphogenetic protein-2 (rhBMP-2). *Journal of Medical and Dental Sciences.* 1997: 44: 53–62.

87) **Asahina I, Watanabe M, Sakurai N, Mori M, Enomoto S.** Repair of bone defect in primate mandible using a bone morphogenetic protein (BMP)–hydroxyapatite–collagen composite. *Journal of Medical and Dental Sciences.* 1997: 44: 63–70.

88) **Kenley R, Marden L, Turek T, Jin L, Ron E, Hollinger JO.** Osseous regeneration in the rat calvarium using novel delivery systems for recombinant human bone morphogenetic protein-2 (rhBMP- 2). *Journal of Biomedical Materials and Research.* 1994: 28: 1139–1147.

89) **Kuboki Y, Takita H, Kobayashi D, Tsuruga E, Ohgushi H.** BMP-induced osteogenesis on the surface of hydroxyapatite with geometrically feasible and

nonfeasible structures: topology of osteogenesis. *Journal of Biomedical Materials and Research.* 1998: 39: 190–199.

90) **Sigurdsson TJ, Nygaard L, Tatakis DN, Fu E, Turek TJ, Jin L, Wozney JM, Wikesjo UM.** Periodontal repair in dogs: evaluation of rhBMP-2 carriers. *Int J Periodontol and Rest Dent.* 1996: 16: 524–537.

91) **Saito N, Takaoka K.** New synthetic biodegradable polymers as BMP carriers for bone tissue engineering. *Biomaterials.* 2003: 24: 2287–2293.

92) **Miyamoto S, Takaoka K, Okada T et al.** Evaluation of polylactic acid homopolymers as carriers for bone morphogenetic protein. *Clin Orthop Relat Res.* 1992: 278: 274–285.

93) **Saito N, Okada T, Horiuchi H.** Local bone formation by injection of recombinant human bone morphogenetic protein-2 contained in polymer carriers. *Bone.* 2003: 32: 381–386.

94) **Matsushita N, Terai H, Okada T et al.** A new bone-inducing biodegradable porous beta-tricalcium phosphate. *J Biomed Mater Res.* 2004: 70: 450–458.

95) **Kaito T, Myoui A, Takaoka K et al.** Potentiation of the activity of bone morphogenetic protein-2 in bone regeneration by a PLA–PEG/hydroxyapatite composite. *Biomaterials.* 2005: 26: 73–79.

96) **Winet H, Hollinger JO.** Incorporation of poly-lactide-poly-glycolide in a cortical defect: neoosteogenesis in a bone chamber. *J Biomed Mater Res.* 1993: 27: 667–676.

97) **Mayer M, Hollinger J, Ron E et al.** Maxillary alveolar cleft repair in dogs using recombinant human bone morphogenetic protein-2 and a polymer carrier. *Plast Reconstr Surg.* 1996: 98: 247–259.

98) **Kokubo S, Fujimoto R, Yokota S et al.** Bone regeneration by recombinant human bone morphogenetic protein-2 and a novel biodegradable carrier in a rabbit ulnar defect model. *Biomaterials.* 2003: 24: 1643–1651.

99) **Kawamoto T, Motohashi N, Kitamura A** *et al.* Experimental tooth movement into bone induced by recombinant human bone morphogenetic protein-2. *Cleft Palate Craniofac J.* 2003: 40: 538–543.

100) **Hu JJ, Jin D, Quan DP** et al. Bone defect repair with a new tissue-engineered bone carrying bone morphogenetic protein in rabbits. *Di Yi Jun Yi Da Xue Xue Bao.* 2005: 25: 1369-1374.

101) **Jeon O, Song SJ, Kang SW** *et al.* Enhancement of ectopic bone formation by bone morphogenetic protein-2 released from a heparin-conjugated poly-lactic-co-glycolic acid) scaffold. *Biomaterials.* 2005: 28: 2763–2771.

102) **Lutolf MP, Lauer-Fields JL, Schmoekel HG** *et al.* Synthetic matrix metalloproteinase-sensitive hydrogels for the conduction of tissue regeneration: engineering cell-invasion characteristics. *Proc Natl Acad Sci USA.* 2003: 100: 5413–5418.

103) **Pratt AB, Weber FE, Schmoekel HG** *et al.* Synthetic extracellular matrices for *in situ* tissue engineering. *Biotechnol Bioeng.* 2004: 86: 27–36.

104) **Geiger M, Li RH, Friess W.** Collagen sponges for bone regeneration with rhBMP-2. *Adv Drug Deliv Rev.* 2003: 55: 1613–1629.

105) **Kirker-Head CA.** Potential applications and delivery strategies for bone morphogenetic proteins. *Adv Drug Deliv Rev.* 2000: 43: 65–92.

106) **Gautschi OP, Frey SP, Zellweger R.** Bone morphogenetic proteins in clinical applications. *NZ J Surg.* 2007: 77: 626–631.

107) **Yang C, Hillas PJ, Baez JA** *et al.* The application of recombinant human collagen in tissue engineering. *BioDrugs.* 2004: 18: 103–119.

108) **Mano J, Reis RL.** Osteochondral defects: present situation and tissue engineering approaches. *J Tissue Eng Regen Med.* 2007: 1: 261–273.

109) **Malafaya PB, Gomes ME, Salgado AJ** *et al.* Polymer based scaffolds and carriers for bioactive agents from different natural origin materials. *Adv Exp Med Biol.* 2003: 534: 201–233.

110) **Prabaharan M, Mano JF.** Chitosan-based particles as controlled drug delivery systems. *Drug Deliv.* 2005: 12: 41–57.

111) **Liang D, Zuo A, Wang B et al.** *In vitro* osteogenesis of the compound of chitosan and recombinant human bone morphogenetic protein 2. *Zhongguo Xiu Fu Chong Jian Wai Ke Za Zhi.* 2005: 19: 721–724.

112) **Hsieh CY, Hsieh HJ, Liu HC et al.** Fabrication and release behaviour of a novel freeze-gelled chitosan -PGA scaffold as a carrier for rhBMP-2. *Dent Mater.* 2006: 22: 622–629.

113) **Lopez-Lacomba JL, Garcia-Cantalejo JM, Casado JVS et al.** Use of rhBMP-2 activated chitosan films to improve osseointegration. *Biomacromolecules.* 2006: 7: 792–798.

114) **Hattori T.** Experimental investigations of osteogenesis and chondrogenesis by implant of BMP–fibrin glue mixture. *Nippon Seikeigeka Gakkai Zasshi.* 1990: 64: 824–834.

115) **Patel VV, Zhao L, Wong P et al.** Controlling bone morphogenetic protein diffusion and bone morphogenetic protein stimulated bone growth using fibrin glue. *Spine.* 2006: 31: 1201–1206.

116) **Smith JD, Melhem ME, Magge KT et al.** Improved growth factor directed vascularization into fibrin constructs through inclusion of additional extracellular molecules. *Microvasc Res.* 2007: 73: 84–94.

117) **Arnander C, Westermark A, Veltheim R et al.** Three dimensional technology and bone morphogenetic protein in frontal bone reconstruction. *J Craniofac Surg.* 2006: 17: 275–279.

118) **Kim HD, Valentini RF.** Retention and activity of BMP-2 in hyaluronic acid-based scaffolds *in vitro*. *J Biomed Mater Res.* 2002: 59: 573–584.

119) **Kim J, Kim IS, Cho TH et al.** Bone regeneration using hyaluronic acid-based hydrogel with bone morphogenic protein-2 and human mesenchymal stem cells. *Biomaterials.* 2007: 28: 1830–1837.

120) **Zou X, Li H, Chen L.** Stimulation of porcine bone marrow stromal cells by hyaluronan, dexamethasone and rhBMP-2. *Biomaterials.* 2004: 25: 5375–5385.

121) **Chen FM, Zhao YM, Zhang R.** Periodontal regeneration using novel glycidyl methacrylated dextran (Dex- GMA)/gelatin scaffolds containing microspheres loaded with bone morphogenetic proteins. *J Control Release.* 2007: 121: 81–90.

122) **Maire M, Chaubet F, Mary P.** Bovine BMP osteoinductive potential enhanced by functionalized dextran-derived hydrogels. *Biomaterials.* 2005: 26: 5085–5092.

123) **Karageorgiou V, Meinel L, Hofmann S** *et al.* Bone morphogenetic protein-2 decorated silk fibroin films induce osteogenic differentiation of human bone marrow stromal cells. *J Biomed Mater Res.* 2004: 71: 528–537.

124) **Li C, Vepari C, Jin HJ.** Electrospun silk-BMP-2 scaffolds for bone tissue engineering. *Biomaterials.* 2006: 27: 3115–3124.

125) **Meinel L, Karageorgiou V, Hofmann S.** Engineering bone-like tissue *in vitro* using human bone marrow stem cells and silk scaffolds. *J Biomed Mater Res A.* 2004: 71: 25–34.

126) **Tsuruga E, Takita H, Itoh H.** Pore size of porous hydroxyapatite as the cell-substratum controls BMP-induced osteogenesis. *J Biochem.* 1997: 121: 317–324.

127) **Saitoh H, Takata T, Nikai H.** Effect of polylactic acid on osteoinduction of demineralized bone: preliminary study of the usefulness of polylactic acid as a carrier of bone morphogenetic protein. *J Oral Rehabil.* 1994: 21: 431–438.

128) **Gepstein R, Weiss RE, Hallel T.** Bridging large defects in bone by demineralized bone matrix in the form of a powder. A radiographic, histological, and radioisotope-uptake study in rats. *Journal of Bone and Joint Surgery, American Volume.* 1987: 69: 984–992.

129) **Einhorn TA, Lane JM, Burstein AH, Kopman CR, Vigorita VJ**. The healing of segmental bone defects induced by demineralised bone matrix. A radiographic and biomechanical study. *Journal of Bone and Joint Surgery, American Volume*. 1984: 66: 274–279.

130) **Becker W, Schenk R, Higuchi K, Lekholm U, Becker BE**. Variations in bone regeneration adjacent to implants augmented with barrier membranes alone or with demineralized freeze– dried bone or autologous grafts: a study in dogs. *Int J Oral and Maxil Imp*. 1995: 10: 143–154.

131) **BeckerW, Lynch SE, Lekholm U, Becker BE, Caffesse R, Donath K, Sanchez R**. A comparison of ePTFE membranes alone or in combination with platelet-derived growth factors and insulin like growth factor-I or demineralized freeze–dried bone in promoting bone formation around immediate extraction socket implants. *J Periodontol*. 1992: 63: 929–940.

132) **Strates BS, Tiedeman JJ**. Contribution of osteoinductive and osteoconductive properties of demineralized bone matrix to skeletal repair. *European Journal of Experimental Musculoskeletal Research*. 1993: 2: 61–67.

133) **Ripamonti U, Magan A, Ma S, Van den Heever B, Moehl T, Reddi AH**. Xenogeneic osteogenin, a bone morphogenetic protein, and demineralized bone matrices, including human, induce bone differentiation in athymic rats and baboons. *Matrix*. 1991: 11: 404–411.

134) **Aspenberg P, Wang E, Thorngren KG**. Bone morphogenetic protein induces bone in the squirrel monkey, but bone matrix does not. *Acta Orthop Scand*. 1992: 63: 619–622.

135) **Johnson EE, Urist MR & Finerman GA**. Resistant non-unions and partial or complete segmental defects of long bones. Treatment with implants of a composite of human bone morphogenetic protein (BMP) and autolyzed, antigen-extracted, allogeneic (AAA) bone. *Clinical Orthopaedics and Related Research*. 1992: 277: 229–237.

136) **Johnson EE, Urist MR.** One-stage lengthening of femoral nonunion augmented with human bone morphogenetic protein. *Clinical Orthopaedics and Related Research.* 1998: 347: 105–116.

137) **Celeste AJ, Song JJ, Cox K, Rosen V, Wozney JM.** Bone morphogenetic protein-9, a new member of the TGF beta superfamily. *Journal of Bone and Mineral Research.* 1994: 9: 136.

138) **Celeste AJ, Ross JL, Yamaji N & Wozney JM.** The molecular cloning of human bone morphogenetic proteins-10, 11 and 12, three new members of the transforming growth factor-superfamily. *Journal of Bone and Mineral Research.* 1995: 10: S-336.

139) **Takuwa Y, Ohse C, Wang EA, Wozney JM, Yamashita K.** Bone morphogenetic protein-2 stimulates alkaline phosphatise activity and collagen synthesis in cultured osteoblastic cells. *Biochemical and Biophysical Research Communications.* 1991: 174: 96–101.

140) **Asahina I, Sampath TK, Nishimura I, Hauschka PV.** Human osteogenic protein-1 induces both chondroblastic and osteoblastic differentiation of osteoprogenitor cells derived from newborn rat calvaria. *Journal of Cellular Biology.* 1993: 123: 921–933.

141) **Knutsen R, Wergedal JE, Sampath TK, Baylink DJ, Mohan S.** Osteogenic protein-1 stimulates proliferation and differentiation of human bone cells *in vitro*. *Biochem and Biophy Res Comm.* 1993: 194: 1352–1358.

142) **Maycr H, Scutt AM, Ankenbauer T.** Subtle differences in the mitogenic effects of recombinant human bone morphogenetic proteins-2 to -7 on DNA synthesis in primary bone-forming cells and identification of BMP-2/4 receptor. *Calcified Tissue International.* 1996: 58: 249–255.

143) **Kretzschmar M, Massague J.** SMADs: mediators and regulators of TGF-β signalling. *Current Opinion in Genetics and Development.* 1998: 8: 103–111.

144) **Baker JC, Harland RM.** From receptor to nucleus: the Smad pathway. *Current Opinion in Genetics and Development.* 1997: **7**: 467–473.

145) **Padgett RW, Cho SH, Evangelista C.** Smads are the central component in transforming growth factor-β signalling. *Pharmacology and Therapeutics.* 1998: 78: 47–52.

146) **Graff JM, Bansal A, Melton DA.** *Xenopus* Mad proteins transducer distinct subsets of signals for the TGF β superfamily. *Cell.* 1996: 85: 479–487.

147) **Luyten FP, Cunningham NS, Ma S, Muthukumaran N, Hammonds RG, Woods WI, Reddi AH.** Purification and partial amino acid sequence of osteogenin, a protein initiating bone differentiation. *J Biol Chem.* 1989: 264: 13377–13380.

148) **Ripamonti U.** Soluble osteogenic molecular signals and the induction of bone formation. *Biomaterials* 2006: 27: 807–822.

149) **Ripamonti U, Crooks J, Teare J, Petit JC, Rueger DC.** Periodontal tissue regeneration by recombinant human osteogenic protein-1 in periodontally induced furcation defects of the primate Papio ursinus. *S Afr J Sci.* 2002: 98: 361–368.

150) **Ripamonti U, Ramoshebi LN, Patton J, Matsaba T, Teare J, Renton L.** Soluble signals and insoluble substrata: novel molecular cues instructing the induction of bone. In: Massaro EJ, Rogers JM, editors. The skeleton. Totowa, New Jersey: Humana Press, 2004: 15: 217–227.

151) **Vlodavsky I, Folkman J, Sullivan R, Fridman R, Sasse J, Klagsbrun M.** Endothelial cell-derived basic fibroblast growth factor: synthesis and deposition into subendothelial extracellular matrix. *Proc Natl Acad Sci USA* 1987: 84: 2292–2296.

152) **Aberg T, Wozney J, Thesleff I.** Expression patterns of bone morphogenetic proteins (Bmps) in the developing mouse tooth suggest roles in morphogenesis and cell differentiation. *Dev Dyn.*1997: 210: 383–396.

153) **Thomadakis G, Ramoshebi LN, Crooks J, Rueger CD, Ripamonti U.** Immunolocalization of bone morphogenetic protein 2 and 3 and osteogenic

protein-1 during murine tooth root morphogenesis and in other craniofacial structures. *Eur J Oral Sci.* 1999: 107: 368–377.

154) **Thesleff I, Sharpe P**. Signalling networks regulating dental development. *Mech Dev* 1997: 67: 111–123.

155) **Reddi AH**. Morphogenesis and tissue engineering of bone and cartilage: inductive signals, stem cells, and biomimetic biomaterials. *Tissue Eng.* 2001: 6: 351–359.

156) **Seo BM, Miura M, Gronthos S, Bartold PM, Batouli S, Brahin J, Robey PG, Wang CY**. Investigation of multipotent postnatal stem cells from human periodontal ligament. *Lancet.* 2004: 364: 149–155.

157) **Ripamonti U, Heliotis M, Rueger DC, Sampath TK**. Induction of cementogenesis by recombinant human osteogenic protein-1 (hOP-1/BMP-7) in the baboon. *Arch Oral Biol.* 1996: 41: 121–126.

158) **Ripamonti U, Heliotis M, Rueger DC, Sampath TK**. Induction of cementogenesis by recombinant human osteogenic protein-1 (hOP-1/BMP-7) in the baboon. *Arch Oral Biol.* 1996: 41: 121–126.

159) **Nyman S, Lindhe J, Karring T, Rylander H**. New attachment following surgical treatment of human periodontal disease. *J Clin Periodontol.* 1982: 4: 290–296.

160) **Wikesjo UM, Selvig KA, Zimmerman G, Nilveus R**. Periodontal repair in dogs: healing in experimentally created chronic periodontal defects. *J Periodontol.* 1991: 62: 258–263.

161) **Huang KK, Shen C, Chiang CY, Hsieh YD, Fu E**. Effects of bone morphogenetic protein-6 on periodontal wound healing in a fenestration defect of rats. *J Periodontal Res.* 2005: 40: 1–10.

162) **Wikesjo UME, Sorenson RG, Kinoshita A, Li J, Wozney JM**. Effect of recombinant human bone morphogenetic protein - 12 (rhBMP-12) on regeneration of alveolar bone and periodontal attachment. *J Clin Periodontol.* 2004: 31: 662–670.

163) **Sorensen RG, Polimeni G, Kinoshita A, Wozney JM, Wikesjo UME.** Effect of recombinant human bone morphogenetic protein-12 (rhBMP-12) on regeneration of periodontal attachment following tooth implantation in dogs. *J Clin Periodontol.* 2004: 31: 654–661.

164) **Marden LJ, Hollinger JO, Chaudhari A, Turek T, Schaub RG, Ron E.** Recombinant human bone morphogenetic protein-2 is superior to demineralized bone matrix in repairing craniotomy defects in rats. *Journal of Biomedical Materials Research.* 1994: 28: 1127–1138.

165) **Yasko AW, Lane JM, Fellinger EJ, Rosen V, Wozney JM, Wang EA.** The healing of segmental bone defects, induced by recombinant human bone morphogenetic protein (rhBMP-2). A radiographic, histological, and biomechanical study in rats. *Journal of Bone and Joint Surgery American Volume.* 1992: 74: 659–670.

166) **Kirker-Head CA, Gerhart TN, Schelling SH, Hennig GE, Wang E, Holtrop ME.** Long-term healing of bone using recombinant human bone morphogenetic protein 2. *Clinical Orthopaedics and Related Research.* 1995: 318: 222–230.

167) **Toriumi DM, Kotler HS, Luxenberg DP, Holtrop ME, Wang EA.** Mandibular reconstruction with a recombinant bone-inducing factor. Functional, histologic, and biomechanical evaluation. *Archives of Otolaryngology: Head and Neck Surgery.* 1991: 117: 1101–1112.

168) **Sandhu HS, Kanim LE, Kabo JM, Toth JM, Zeegen EN, Liu D, Delamarter RB, Dawson EG.** Effective doses of recombinant human bone morphogenetic protein-2 in experimental spinal fusion. *Spine.* 1996: 21: 2115–2122.

169) **Zegzula HD, Buck DC, Brekke J, Wozney JM, Hollinger JO.** Bone formation with use of rhBMP-2 (recombinant human bone morphogenetic protein-2). *Journal of Bone and Joint Surgery, American Volume.* 1997: 79: 1778–1790.

170) **Lee SC, Shea M, Battle MA, Kozitza K, Ron E, Turek T, Hayes WC.** Healing of large segmental defects in rat femurs is aided by RhBMP-2 in PLGA matrix. *Journal of Biomedical Materials Research.* 1994: 28: 1149–1156.

171) **Cook SD, Baffes GC, Wolfe MW, Sampath TK, Rueger DC.** The effect of recombinant human osteogenic protein-1 on healing of large segmental bone defects. *Journal of Bone and Joint Surgery.* 1994: 76: 827–838.

172) **Cook SD, Baffes GC, Wolfe MW, Sampath TK, Rueger DC.** Recombinant human bone morphogenetic protein-7 induces healing in a canine long-bone segmental defect model. *Clinical Orthopaedics and Related Research.* 1994: 301: 302–312.

173) **Stevenson S, Cunningham N, Toth J, Davy D, Reddi AH.** The effect of osteogenin (a bone morphogenetic protein) on the formation of bone in orthotopic segmental defects in rats. *Journal of Bone and Joint Surgery, American Volume.* 1994: 76: 1676–1687.

174) **Marglin MD, Cogan AG, Taylor M, Buck D, McAllister TN, Toth C & McAllister B.** Maxillary sinus augmentation in the non-human primate: a comparative radiographic and histologic study between recombinant human osteogenic protein1 and natural bone mineral. *J Periodontol.* 1998: 69: 911–919.

175) **Nevins M, Kirker-Head C, Nevins M, Wozney JA, Palmer R, Graham D.** Bone formation in the goat maxillary sinus induced by absorbable collagen sponge implants impregnated with recombinant human bone morphogenetic protein-2. *Int J Periodontol and Rest Dent.* 1996: 16: 8–19.

176) **Boyne PJ, Marx RE, Nevins M, Triplett G, Lazaro E, Lilly LC, Alder M, Nummikoski P.** A feasibility study evaluating rhBMP-2/ absorbable collagen sponge for maxillary sinus floor augmentation. *International Journal of Periodontics and Restorative Dentistry.* 1997: 17: 10–25.

177) **Howell TH, Fiorellini J, Jones A, Alder M, Nummikoski P, Lazaro M, Lilly L, Cochran D.** A feasibility study evaluating rhBMP- 2/absorbable collagen sponge device for local alveolar ridge preservation or augmentation. *Int J Periodontol and Rest Dent.* 1997: 17: 125–139.

178) **Groeneveld HHJ, Bruggenkate CM, Tuinzing DB, Burger EH.** Histomorphometrical analysis of bone formed in human maxillary sinus floor elevations grafted with OP-1 device, demineralized bone matrix or autogenous bone. Comparison with non-grafted sites in a series of case reports. *Clinical Oral Implants Research* 1999: 10(6): 499-509.

179) **Geesink RGT, Hoefnagels NHM, Bulstra SK.** Osteogenic activity of OP-1, bone morphogenetic protein-7 (BMP-7), in a human fibular defect model. *Journal of Bone and Joint Surgery, British Volume.* 1999: 81: 710–718.

180) **Torimi DM, Kotler HS, Luxenberg DP, Holtrop ME, Wang EA.** Mandibular reconstruction with a recombinant bone-inducing factor. Functional, histologic, and biomechanical evaluation. *Arch Otolaryngol Head Neck Surg.* 1991: 117: 1101-1112.

181) **Boyne PJ.** Animal studies of application of rhBMP-2 in maxillofacial reconstruction. *Bone.* 1996: 19: 83-92.

182) **Giannobile WV, Ryan S, Shih MS, Su DL, Kaplan PL, Chan TC.** Recombinant human osteogenic protein-1(OP-1) stimulates periodontal wound healing in Class III furcation defects. *J Periodontol.* 1998: 69: 129-137.

183) **Kinoshita A, Oda S, Takahashi K, Yokota S, Ishikawa I.** Periodontal regeneration by application of recombinant human bone morphogenetic protein-2 to horizontal circumferential defects created by experimental periodontitis in beagle dogs. *J Periodontol.* 1997: 68: 103-109.

184) **Cochran DL, Schenk R, Buser D, Wozney JM, Jones AA.** Recombinant human bone morphogenetic protein-2 stimulation of bone formation around endosseous dental implants. *J Periodontol.* 1999: 70: 139-150.

185) **Sailer HF, Kolb E.** Application of purified bone morphogenetic protein (BMP) in cranio-maxillo-facial surgery. BMP in compromised surgical reconstructions using titanium implants. *J Cranio Max Fac Surg*. 1994: 22: 2-11.

186) **Khan SN, Sandhu HS, Lane JM, Cammisa FP, Girardi FP.** Bone morphogenetic proteins: relevance in spine surgery. *Orthop Clin North Am.* 2002: 33: 447–463.

187) **Damien CJ, Grob D, Boden SD, Benedict JJ.** Purified bovine BMP extract and collagen for spine arthrodesis: preclinical safety and efficacy. *Spine*. 2002: 27: S50–S58.

188) **Schellekens H.** Immunogenicity of therapeutic proteins: clinical implications and future prospects. *Clin Ther*. 2002: 24: 1720–1740.

189) **Schellekens H.** Immunogenicity of therapeutic proteins. *Nephrol Dial Transplant*. 2003: 18: 1257–1259.

190) **Poynton AR, Lane JM.** Safety profile for the clinical use of bone morphogenetic proteins in the spine. *Spine*. 2002: 27: S40–S48.

191) **Walker DH, Wright NM.** Bone morphogenetic proteins and spinal fusion. *Neurosurg Focus*. 2002: 13: E370.

192) **Carreon LY, Glassman SD, Dimar JR, Puno RM, Campbell MJ.** Adverse events in patients re-exposed to bone morphogenetic protein for spine surgery. *Spine*. 2008: 33: 391–393.

193) **Westerhuis RJ, Bezooijen RL, Kloen P.** Use of BMP in traumatology. *Injury-International Journal of the Care of the Injured*. 2005: 36: 1405–1412.

194) **McKay WF, Peckham SM, Badura JM.** A comprehensive clinical review of rh bone morphogenetic protein-2. *Int Orthop*. 2007: 31: 6: 729-734.

195) **White AP, Vaccaro AR, Hall JA.** Clinical applications of BMP-7/OP-1 in fractures, non-unions and spinal fusion. *Int Orthop*. 2007: 31(6): 735-41.

196) **Luginbuehl V, Meinel L, Merkle HP.** Localized delivery of growth factors for bone repair. *Eur J Pharm Biopharm*. 2004: 58: 197–208.

197) **Hadjiargyrou M, Lombardo F, Zhao S.** Transcriptional profiling of bone regeneration. Insight into the molecular complexity of wound repair. *J Biol Chem.* 2002: 277: 30177–30182.

198) **Klosch B, Furst W, Kneidinger R.** Expression and purification of biologically active rat bone morphogenetic protein- 4 produced as inclusion bodies in recombinant *Escherichia coli. Biotechnol Lett.* 2005: 27: 1559–1564.

199) **Schmoekel HG, Weber FE, Schense JC.** Bone repair with a form of BMP-2 engineered for incorporation into fibrin cell ingrowth matrices. *Biotechnol Bioeng.* 2005: 89: 253–262.

200) **Bessa PC, Pedro AJ, Klosch B.** Osteoinduction in human fat-derived stem cells by recombinant human bone morphogenetic protein-2 produced in *Escherichia coli. Biotechnol Lett.* 2008: 30(1): 15-21.

201) **Matsumoto A, Yamaji K, Kawanami M, Kato H.** Effect of aging on bone formation induced by recombinant human bone morphogenetic protein-2 combined with fibrous collagen membranes at subperiosteal sites. *J Periodontol Res.* 2000: 36(3): **175 – 182.**

202) **Nakamura T, Yamamoto M, Tamura M, Izumi Y.** Effects of growth / differentiation factor-5 on human periodontal ligament cells. *J Periodontol Res.* 2003: 38(6): 597–605.

203) **Huang KK, Chiang Y, Hsieh YD, Earl Fu.** Effects of bone morphogenetic protein-6 on periodontal wound healing in a fenestration defect of rats. *J Periodontol Res.* 2004: 40(1): **1–10.**

204) **Miyaji H, Sugaya T, Kato K, Kawamura N, Tsuji H, Kawanami M.** Dentin resorption and cementum-like tissue formation by bone morphogenetic protein application. *J Periodontol Res.* 2005: 41(4): **311 – 315.**

205) **Yoshimoto T, Yamamoto M, Kadomatsu H, Sakoda K, Yonamine Y, Yuichi Izumi.** Recombinant human growth/differentiation factor-5 (rhGDF-

5) induced bone formation in murine calvariae. *J Periodontol Res.* 2005: 41(2): **140–147.**

206) **Wikesjo Um, Qahash M, Polimeni G, Susin C, Richard H.** Alveolar ridge augmentation using implants coated with recombinant human bone morphogenetic protein-2: histologic observations. *Journal of Clinical Periodontology.* 2008: 35(11): 1001–1010.

207) **Jovanovic SA, Hunt DR, Bernard GW, Spiekermann H, Wozney JM.** Bone reconstruction following implantation of rhBMP-2 and guided bone regeneration in canine alveolar ridge defects. *Clin Oral Implants Res.* 2007: 18(2): 224-30.

208) **Pang EK, Kim CS, Choi SH, Chai JK, Kim CK, Han SB, Cho KS.** Effect of recombinant human bone morphogenetic protein-4 dose on bone formation in a rat calvarial defect model. *J Periodontol.* 2004: 75(10): 1364-70.

209) **Yashiro R, Nagasawa T, Kiji M, Hormdee D, Kobayashi H, Koshy G.** Transforming growth factor-β stimulates Interleukin-11 production by human periodontal ligament and gingival fibroblasts. *Journal of Clinical Periodontology.* 2008: 33(3): **165 – 171.**

210) **Sieber C, Kopf J, Hiepen C, Knaus P.** Recent advances in BMP receptor signalling. *Cytokine Growth Factor Rev.* 2009: 20(5): 343-355.

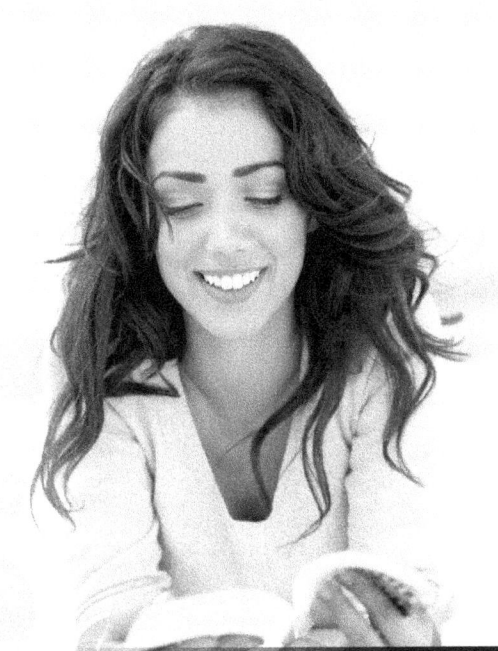

i want morebooks!

Buy your books fast and straightforward online - at one of world's fastest growing online book stores! Environmentally sound due to Print-on-Demand technologies.

Buy your books online at
www.get-morebooks.com

Kaufen Sie Ihre Bücher schnell und unkompliziert online – auf einer der am schnellsten wachsenden Buchhandelsplattformen weltweit! Dank Print-On-Demand umwelt- und ressourcenschonend produziert.

Bücher schneller online kaufen
www.morebooks.de

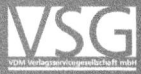

VDM Verlagsservicegesellschaft mbH
Heinrich-Böcking-Str. 6-8
D - 66121 Saarbrücken

Telefon: +49 681 3720 174
Telefax: +49 681 3720 1749

info@vdm-vsg.de
www.vdm-vsg.de

Lightning Source UK Ltd.
Milton Keynes UK
UKHW011006150421
382040UK00001B/119